YEAST CONTROL

IN

SEVEN DAYS

How to Rebuild Health and Control Candida
New Expanded Edition

by

S. A. D'Onofrio, D.N., D.D.

Artwork by Mitch Couasnon

Published in the Republic of the United States of America

ISBN 0-9709769-0-9

FirstEdition   1990
SecondEdition 1995
ThirdEdition   2001

TABLE OF CONTENTS

PART ONE

PART TWO
THE PROGRAMS

ACKNOWLEDGMENTS

I acknowledge and thank God for the Divine inspiration when it came through, the Energies needed to complete this project and the Entities sent to guide me.

I thank all my teachers, past, present and future for their caring, patience, understanding and instructions, verbal and written: Bing Escudera, Dr. Benito Reyes, Dr. Anne Mitchell, Dr. Robert Bradford, Dr. Kevin Kopriva, Dr. Gary Martin, Dr. Mike Kelley, Tom Lord, my parents, friends and antagonists for their lessons.

I especially thank Christina Calderone for her tireless editing and inspiration through difficult passages. The ease of reading and the ability to understand many difficult parts of this work is due largely to her suggestions. Bless you.

I thank Barbara Lolli and Pamela Mullenix, without whose computer skills I would still be typing.

I thank Chuck Hamil for computer technical support.

I thank Mitch Couasnon for seeing the ideas in my mind and getting them down on paper.

I thank Sandra Louise Hart for her love and support through the hard times.

NOTICE

This program is designed to aid the doctor or consultant in the nutritional counseling and education of the patient in sound nutritional principles. The suggested foods, supplements, recommendations and procedures are to be used by the doctor or consultant based upon his or her professional knowledge and judgment.

No statement contained herein shall be construed as a claim or representation of use in the diagnosis, cure, mitigation, treatment or prevention of any disease or condition.

These nutritional programs, food supplements, and suggestions are not drugs, nor are they intended to replace any drug, manipulation, or physical therapy, and/or any medical procedure which may be deemed necessary or indicated by a medical doctor.

The results of this program are nutritional only and may differ depending upon the individual.

The quality of your life and ability to pursue happiness are dependent on your liberty to choose wellness over illness. The constitution of the United States of America validates your God given right to choose. Your body is the temple of God. It is your inalienable right and responsibility to maintain the wellness and vitality of this temple to carry out your divine purpose in this world.

IN MEMORIAM

To the memory of Dr. Paavo Airola, N.D., whose example and books taught me how to "Be Well", and for the inspiration to become a natural health practitioner. Thank you.

"An invitation to a sensation"

S*A*I*O*E

....ultimate state of being

It has been estimated that 75% of what you know about living was learned by age three, even before you could talk. We accomplished this through our senses, especially our sixth sense of intuitiion.

Intuition is primarily a feminine function because the pineal gland, the gland of sensory telecommunication, is one third larger in females than most men. Hence women learn faster than men, develope larger brain systems (the corpus collosum) for processing more information between lobes at once and thus trust their sense of intuition, more than men do. It is conceptual thought, gleaned in an instant.

The pineal gland is essential for conceptual thought. When a musician or a poet hears a song, it is first experienced (sensed) as a total concept. Writing it down and scoring it is a secondary analytical thought, primarily a male cerebral function of linear thought.

Linear thought is better for tracking game and bringing home the food. Women being smart, mated with those who could provide and propagate the species. Those who were too sensitive to kill and brought home flowers did not get to add much to the gene pool.

Zen teaches us that if a thought can be spoken, it's essence is not that. Why? Because something is always lost in the translation. But a thought, once transmitted, cannot be altered nor stopped. Neither can an idea. An idea is one of the strongest forces on this plane of existence. Once an idea is formed, concentrated on and projected, it can be sensed by yourself and other sensitive people. A sensitive child thus learns and adopts the ideas of its parents, for survival. A sensation cannot be adequately described by words, tasted, heard, or held. But it can often be powerfully perceived, as in a "sense of health". **Our senses are our earliest learning tools.** In some of us, thought numbed and long forgotten, our senses are still here to serve us.

Health is Peace Within. If you are not at Peace, you are not at ease. You are at dis-ease or ill at ease. Health is a state of Be-ingness. The essence of health can be sensed by one possessing it. It can be sensed by others through their pineal gland. You see, we are all thus connected by this gland's function. There is no Separation of Any of God's Parts.

Using S*A*I*O*E to build Health

We can use **S*A*I*O*E** to gain and maintain our health precisely because it is an invitation to use our best learning tools, our senses. Where to start? A concept can be entered at any point since it has no beginning or end, so we may use this in a circular concept as well as linear.

S- *sense of*
A- *appreciation*
I- *inspiration*
O- *openness*
E- *essence*

sense of   *appreciation*

Health

inspiration   *openness*

essence

An Idea is Mindfulness of a Sensation.(a S*A*I*O*E of Health)
S*A*I*O*E is a Sensation of Mindfulness (an Idea that is sensed)

In order to get a **S**ense of something, e.g.,. your Health, you must **A**ppreciate the values of the concept, be **I**nspired by the dream for energy, be **O**pen to it as *already happening* and be able to distill the **E**ssence of the idea as simply as possible. Just as numbers are labels or outpictures for a concept, it is important to outpicture the concept of your end result in order to bring you back to a sense of it. **SAIOE**

SAIOE can be used to create anything your imagination can see. For further information on seminars, workshops and workbooks contact the creator of SAIOE, Robert Heiman, CEO, Epicuren Products at 949-588-5807 or email RHeiman@Epicuren.com.

A folly has been observed that many people waste away their health going after wealth. Then, they spend all their wealth regaining their health. Health may not be everything, but without Health, everything else is not worth very much. Find your*.. **ultimate state of Being.***

A HEALTH GUARDIAN PROGRAM OUTLINE

After many years of refining this program, the latest Health Guardian Program will contain these personalized elements

1. Digestive
   - a. Mastication
   - b. Enzymes
   - c. Food combining

2. Supplementation
3. Internal Cleansing
   - a. Available Modalities
4. Water
   - a. Quantities
   - b. Sources
5. Food
   - a. To Include
   - b. To Avoid
   - c. How To Cook and Prepare
6. Exercise Suggestions
7. Emotional Support
8. Spiritual Encouragement
   - a. Prayer
   - b. Visualization
   - c. S*A*I*O*E.

Of all the elements we mentioned, it has always been my belief, now proven by Science, that your **Spiritual, Mental, and Emotional elements have the greatest effect on your Health and Healing.** There is synergy in combining Spiritual, Mental, Emotional and Physical modalities. I have observed that it has consistently produced far greater and faster results in building Health than trying them one at a time. *Like four tires on your vehicle of life, they all need to be inflated at the same time for best results.* This is best accomplished by using the SAIOE technique, showing you the Essence of your efforts,....
.........*an ultimate state of Being,* Health.

YEAST CONTROL

IN

SEVEN DAYS

How to Rebuild Health and Control Candida
New Expanded Edition

by

S. A. D'Onofrio, D.N., D.D.

Doctorate in Nutripathy
Doctorate in Divinity

Third Edition
Health Guardian Publications

A message from
Health Guardian's Nutripath
Dr. Sal D'Onofrio, DN, DD.

Dear Friends,

Successfully teaching people how to **control** *candida albicans* for over nineteen years is still rewarding. Thank you. At Health Guardians, we are committed to educating individuals to have the skills and confidence needed to take responsibility for personal health concerns. These programs are vehicles for health. They can take you as far as you choose, as fast as you desire and as safely as possible. Control is a Technique, Health is a Journey and Programs are the Vehicles.

Clinical research has proven that antifungal formulas, immune stimulation and new internal cleansing products have greatly enhanced the effectiveness of the *Yeast Control In Seven Days* program. Due to repeated requests, we are including guidelines to our program. (see pages 70, 71, and 72). The DE Formula has added a new dimension.

Our basic philosophy includes: 1. **Cleansing** the body (remove the negative environment which stresses the immune system and that candida needs in order to proliferate). 2. **Building** the body through proper digestion, nutrition and supplementation thus restoring a weakened immune system - one of the *main reasons* for a candida overgrowth. 3. **Control** solutions (regulating the actual candida organisms). 4. **S.A.I.O.E** (Sense of, Appreciation, Inspiration, Openness, Essence)

NOTE - Please keep in mind when reading this book that **Candida is not the problem**, it is a symptom that the **immune system**, which controls candida, is overwhelmed. The immune system usually is NOT receiving the nutrients it needs from the **digestive system**. "Stomach is Mother to All systems of the body". **If your digestion is not working properly, you are not either!**

I invite you to call us and try our guided, step-by-step health building programs. Start feeling better. Just BE IT, DO IT, HAVE IT!!

Be Well,
Dr. Sal D'Onofrio, DN, DD   call us now at: 1-888-231-0738

Chapter One

WHY ANOTHER BOOK?

This book is written as a result of the lack of literature offering a quick, effective, safe and understandable method of dealing with the Candida problem. Most books offer three to twelve months of diet deprivation, misinformation about what can be eaten, and very little on how to deal with the digestive problems, blood sugar imbalances, parasites and concurrent allergies associated with Candidiasis (candida overgrowths).

By addressing these principles, I have been successfully helping clients control Candida overgrowths since 1984. In as little as three to seven days the first relief in years has been reported by sufferers who "have tried everything and nothing worked." Due to <u>biochemical individuality,</u> different programs are offered, see Sources to address the level of tolerance of the individual. Contained are the Seven Day Program and The Seven Day Intensive Program.

For Whom This Book is Intended

This book is intended to help anyone who is interested in self healing through wellness. Wellness comes through education. It is the responsibility of the doctor to teach, and of the client to be willing to learn from all available sources.

I have written this book in layman's language to facilitate the physician in guiding the client through the program on their return to health. **I highly recommend that this program be carried out under the guidance of a qualified health professional. I do not** advise the self- educated client to attempt to deal with this problem alone. At least **enroll a friend** to help.

1

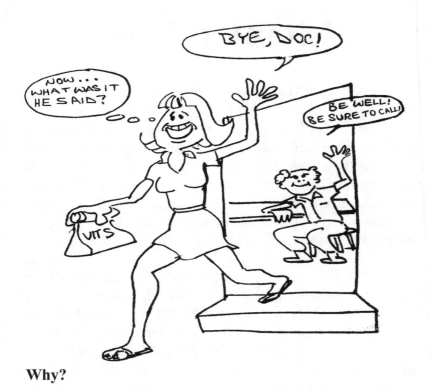

Why?

Because mental confusion is one of the hallmarks of Candidiasis. It has been my experience that many clients have sabotaged this program as a result of this confusion, even with professional advice available.

I have taken an extended program (usually six months to one year), and condensed it to seven days. It must be adhered to closely for best results. Client substitutions have inadvertently sabotaged the program by the inclusion of as little as one item. (See Chapter 13 on "How To Sabotage This Program.")
NOTE-If you want symptomatic relief of Candidiasis, see a medical doctor. For self healing, read on.

Chapter Two

CURES VS. HEALING

The Setup

I believe in wellness through education and that doctors are obliged to teach as well as give remedies. I believe that any attempt to "cure" a disease without altering the personal processes which created the illness is an exercise in self-sabotage through dis-empowerment. On a certain level, we set up our bodies to accommodate pathogens. We do this by creating a body environment which is hospitable for fungal, bacterial and viral pathogens to grow.

Two shiny aluminum garbage pails were bought. One was used in a restaurant kitchen for three months, the other stored in a closet. They were then placed outside in the heat of a summer's day. The pail with food for the flies soon had fly eggs in the decaying matter. The clean pail had nothing on which the flies could exist. They landed and then quickly left in search of a home. If you compare the flies to fungus, virus and bacteria, you may then see the role **you** play in setting up for disease. What does the inside of your body (colon) look like?

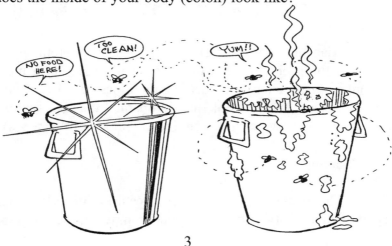

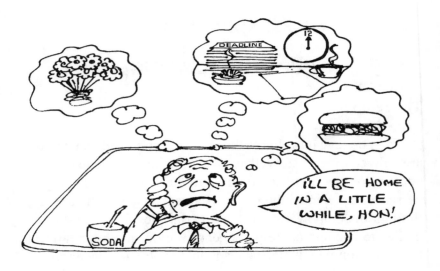

We then create excessive stress from the over use and abuse of life's gifts. Too much food, work, drink or relationship is, simply, too much. This slowly weakens our immune system. This is our part in the process. Once we have weakened ourselves, Nature will take its course. It has to. **Dis-ease is our early warning system and not to be ignored.** It really breaks down to this:

If you do not take the time to be well,
you will take the time to be sick.

Also, just suppressing the symptoms will not remove the cause of the problem. That method usually leads to a more serious problem later on by driving the illness deeper. This is how we set up chronic problems. "Idiopathic" diseases supposedly have no known origin. (Notice the idiocy of this term.)

Real Healing

The level of health is a direct result of lifestyle. When a part of your lifestyle does not support your wellness, it must be

4

changed to produce a different result. I know of no other successful way which promotes health. A cure is a removal of symptoms, and any good doctor is capable of that. A doctor does the coaching, but you do the hard work. After all, it is the whole person we are dealing with, not just the disease.

Real healing is the self care a person does consciously on the spiritual, mental/emotional and physical levels.

Removing pain and suffering is well and good, but it is only half the process. Finding the causes and correctly addressing them is the other half. If this work is not done, return visits to the doctor are inevitable. The cycle of dependency on symptomatic relief (cures) is thus started.

The unwillingness to take responsibility in the creation of disease and the healing of the body continues this cycle of dependency. Believing the story that germs cause disease and only doctors can make you well, feeds directly into the victim/savior roles. This removes responsibility from creating any part in the scenario and takes any credit for getting well away from you. This is most dis-empowering. When it is not stopped, this mindset predisposes you to a lifetime of disease care (symptomatic relief) dependency.

Most of us have been raised in this mindset (The Germ Theory of Disease). It is only a theory, based on partial truths. "The best lie is the closest slice to the truth." It is up to the individual to seek the whole story and be re-educated. Wellness through education teaches that to get different results, you must enroll yourself in different behavior. Since all diseases are "diseases" of lifestyle, **lifestyle modifications are necessary** if you choose to alter any dependency cycles. The choice is yours, the power is yours.

5

Chapter Three

HEAL-THY IMMUNE SYSTEM

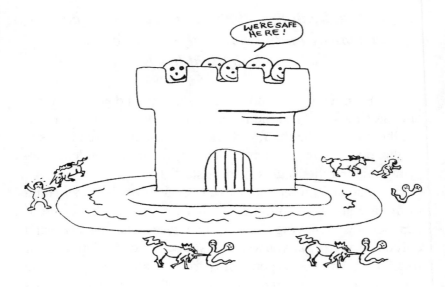

Castle and Moat

It must be stated that the natural protection from any illness is a healthy body and a properly functioning immune system. The two cannot be separated. Like a castle with a moat around it, healthy cells cannot be directly invaded by an attacking virus, bacteria or fungus. While these invaders are looking for a way across the moat, the defenders - **the immune system** - attack and remove the would-be invaders.

Let's say the moat ran dry due to lack of supplying it with the proper substance: water. Or the moat was not cleaned properly and filled up with debris. Now the invaders can easily cross the first line of defense. If the structural integrity of the castle's stone walls are intact, they can hold out until the immune system arrives. Until then, the invaders are laying siege and preventing the supplies needed to keep the walls strong. If the immune system does not show up in time, the invaders' very presence wears down the walls and causes the death of the cells, or worse, a take over, as with viral cancer. All is not yet lost. It is still possible to evict the invaders and return the castle to normal.

You can see that even a healthy cell can be worn down and invaded if the immune system is not there to protect it. Even a damaged cell can be repaired if no further damage continues.

The key to recovery is a healthy immune system.

This cannot be overstated. The continued use of medications is only a temporary cure. As soon as they are discontinued the problem returns. The cause of the depressed immune system must be addressed for real healing to occur. For optimum results in any program, the immune system must be supported and maintained at a high level of efficiency by any and all means available.

Normal Defenses

The primary function of the immune system is to recognize harmful substances to the body, mark them, kill them, and eliminate them.

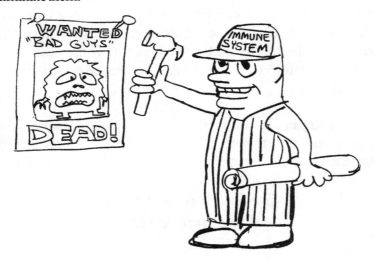

The immune system is comprised of two types of defenders. The various white blood cells, controlled by the Thymus gland are thus called T-Cells. The others are special large proteins, immunoglobulins, which are made in the bone marrow, thus called B-Cells. Each have special jobs. White blood cells flow throughout the body seeking invaders. When they find them, they attack, bind them up, kill and remove them. The large proteins (antibodies) are made in response to the presence of foreign proteins (antigens/allergens) in the blood. They attach themselves to the invading antigens/allergens and mark them for removal from the blood by the white blood cells.

The specific large proteins (Immunoglobulin A) that line and protect the entire mucus lining of the intestinal tract are always present. They keep undigested food molecules from entering the blood by marking them as foreign invaders. If the

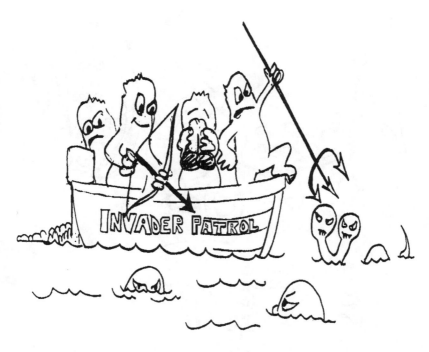

molecule gets by the first immunoglobulin (IgA) and enters the blood, other immunoglobulins, (IgD, IgE, IgG, IgM) are formed in response. **This is why complete protein digestion is essential for a healthy immune system.** When these large proteins are low or not available, partially digested foods can enter the blood and cause an allergic response. This keeps the immune system so busy forming immune complexes and thus removing the unwanted proteins, it doesn't have time to fight the bacterial, viral or fungal invaders.

NOTE- It has been reported that certain experimental infant vacines destroy the Immuno-globulins that line the intestinal tract.

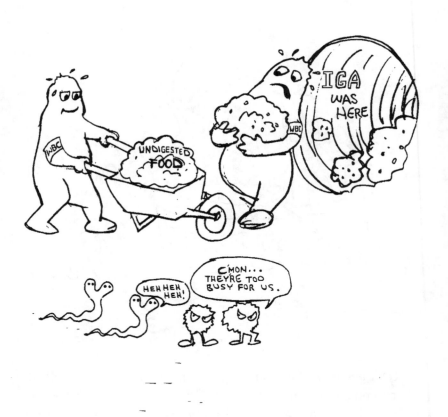

Dr. Aristo Wojdani et al in Clinical Ecology, Volume III, Number 4 states, "Different concentrations of serum immune complexes **blocked the response** of peripheral blood lymphocytes to Candida Albicans as well as the ability of natural Killer cells to lyse tumor target cells." This whole process is very energy consuming and can eventually wear one down to a chronic fatigue syndrome. Epstein Barr virus is often found in candida clients. Allergic reactions also stress the body in other ways (see Chapter 9 on Allergies) causing an overall reduction in available energy. Energy is essential for healthy resistance to invaders and to maintain basic body functions, both of which are a constant in a healthy metabolism.

Chapter Four

CANDIDA ALBICANS

Definition and Symptoms

Candida. What is it? It is a yeast/fungal organism that commonly lives in the mouth, skin, intestinal tract, and vagina. There are several varieties, some are more resistant than others. Antibiotics have no negative effect on candida. (Antibiotics do wipe out friendly bacteria that help suppress candida, and cause it to grow unchecked.) Yeasts are airborne on grasses, grains, fruits, foods, and in drinks. Humans become the host shortly after birth or may have contracted candida from the vaginal canal at birth. Breast-fed babies have a higher resistance to yeasts (if the mother is yeast free) partially due to the lactobacillus bifidus in mother's milk. Bifidus metabolic byproducts kill candida. Cows eat grasses with yeasts, molds and fungi on them which are passed into the milk and are resistant to pasteurization. Bottle-fed infants receive contact to candida from cow's milk, air and foods. Thus, they may contract oral thrush without the immune benefits in bifidus from mother's milk. See the Infant Bottle Formula, page 93.

It is normal to have candida in the system.

Candida in the large intestine is naturally suppressed and controlled by a healthy immune system. It's presence is no immediate threat to a healthy person.

Candidiasis Defined

It is an opportunistic yeast/fungal infection of the skin, oral mucosa, intestinal tract, respiratory tract and vagina caused by the unremoved toxins emitted from an overgrowth of candida albicans.

The amine-like toxins emitted from the candida alkalinize the area, thus decreasing the blood flow to and from the site. This prohibits the arrival of oxygenated blood to the area. Candida is anaerobic. It cannot live in highly oxygenated areas, therefore, it creates an environment that suits its needs. Candida also protects itself by forming immune complexes. Dr. Aristo Wojdani's work shows that these complexes inhibit the response of the immune system to candida. They also block the ability of natural killer cells to attack tumor target cells. The blood flow away from the area is also lessened. This causes a gelation of the area tissues from the buildup of metabolic wastes. The more garbage in the moat, the better for candida to grow in.

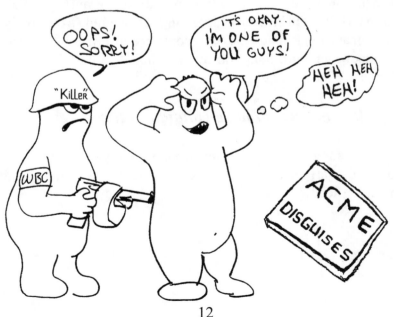

Symptoms and Signs of Candida Overgrowth:

Short term memory loss
Persistent drowsiness
Lack of coordination
Headaches
Mood swings
Loss of balance
Rashes
Mucus in stools
Belching and flatulence
Bad breath
Postnasal drip
Nasal itch and or congestion
Nervous irritability
Tightness of the chest
Dry mouth or throat
Ear sensitivity or fluid in the ears
Heartburn and indigestion

Note: All of the above are usually worse on damp days.

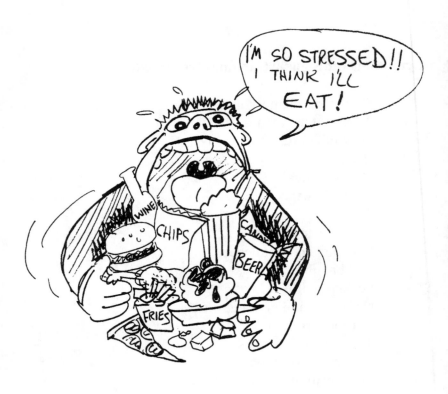

Causes

What causes it? Two conditions must exist. A conducive environment and an instigating pathogen. The overgrowth occurs when the guard, the immune system, is depressed. The immune system normally kills any candida that is not site bound. If candida tries to penetrate the intestine and get into the blood, the healthy immune system will recognize it and kill it. When the immune system is depressed, white blood cells (WBC) may have a suppressed reaction to candida complexes and not attack. Due to a lack of vitamin-C, WBC may not have the ability to move around. They may be overwhelmed by excessive candida and environmental toxins in the blood. The combination of allergic stress on the immune system and certain foods that feed the yeast allows a rapid overgrowth of candida.

14

When the structural integrity of the cell walls are compromised by nutritional deficiencies and the depressed immune system is not removing the invasive candida, then, and only then, will candidiasis occur.

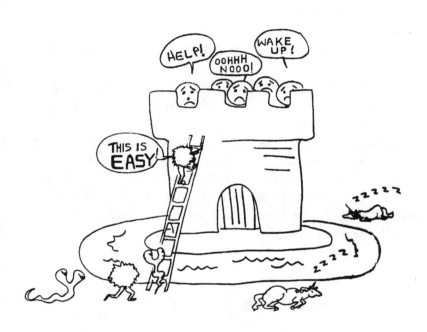

Depressed Immune Function

Depressed immune function can occur when mental, emotional and physical stresses cause a depressed digestive system. Consequently, the main nutrients needed for a healthy, viable, white blood cell, (vitamin-C for leukocyte chemotaxis* and proteins for immunoglobulins) are lacking.

 * Chemotaxis is the WBCs' ability to move to where they are needed.

This is also the case in poor dietary practices which cause high alkalinity; thus, poor absorption of nutrients and poor elimination. A slow moving bowel becomes alkaline, a favorite environment for candida.

Cortisone, aspirin, hormones in foods, hormones in medicine, fluoride in water and toothpaste, mercury from fillings, lead, drugs and other chemicals suppress the immune system. Allergic substances in the body, once handled by the healthy immune system, now go unchecked, creating more stress and additional alkalinity.

Overgrowth also occurs when the other friendly occupants of the environment e.g. lactobacillus acidophilus, are diminished or wiped out. Antibiotics fed to penned livestock enter the food chain thus producing low levels of antibiotics, another immunosuppressant, in human blood. Additional use of antibiotic therapy destroys friendly bacteria faster than they can be replaced. Candida and acidophilus have similar binding sites in the intestine. The less acidophilus in the intestine, the more sites for candida to grow.

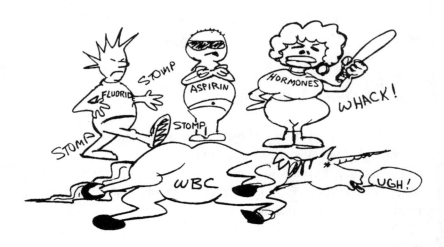

Chapter Five

THE CANCER/CANDIDA CONNECTION

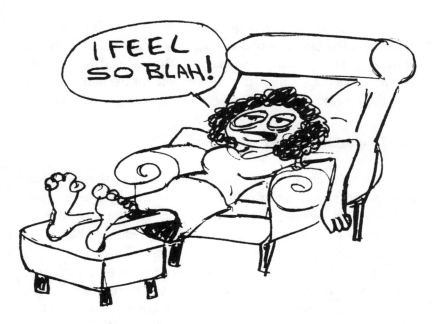

It is known that Candida affects one's behavior and causes physical distress. Many people complain of general discomfort, fatigue, headaches, multiple allergies and high food sensitivities, with depression and unhappiness. Frequently this is due to a Candida overgrowth. The possible seriousness of Candida was once seen on a deeper molecular level.

Dr. William Frederick Koch, M.D., in "Cancer and Its Allied Diseases" 1926, demonstrated that all diseases fall into the same pattern, including every viral and focal infection. The toxins emitted by these infections are the pathogenic agents in metabolic disorders, including toxic goiter and diabetes.

In his book "The Survival Factor in Neoplastic and Viral Disease", Koch identified the atomic groups of the pathogens. These altered the energy producing and energy accepting functions of the cell, the electric dispositions, and the determining bond strengths.

Anoxia: The Determining Factor

William Koch was the first to determine that anoxia, a deficiency of oxygen, was the determining factor in cancer. Mitosis(cell division) is an oxygen mediated pathway. He outlined three specific factors: (1) a disposing factor responsible for the anoxia, (2) an initiating carcinogen, and (3) a supportive or propagative carcinogen.

The Disposing Factor

Koch determined that a disposing factor is fungus, found in all cancer specimens, first identified in 1923 by Glover, again in 1942 by Koch, and in 1948 by Diller, a bacteriologist at the University of Pennsylvania. Koch described the phenomena leading to anoxia. It turns out to be an amine by-product of the fungus, (similar to antibiotic amines widely used in medicine). Chemical amines are carcinogenic for the same reasons. Amines bind the energy producing Functional Carbonyl Group (FCG) of a cell. Efficient oxidation stops and highly inefficient fermentation begins. (Remember an example of rapid oxidation is called fire, and slow oxidation is called rust.)

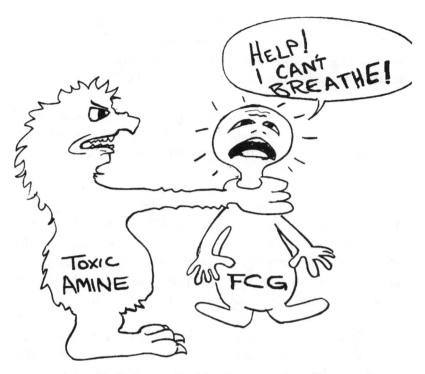

Amines bind the energy producing Functional Carbonyl Group (FCG) of a cell.

Without oxidation to burn up cellular wastes, a toxic buildup inside and outside the cell occurs. This eventually causes a gelation of the tissues in the area (a dirty moat) that predisposes one to cancer. (Dr. Truss, "The Yeast Connnection," cites antibiotic use as a predisposition to Candida, because it also kills the friendly bacteria, acidophilus.) When gelation occurs, the area is deprived of adequate oxygen. Almost all virus, bacteria, and fungus, which are pathogenic to man, are anaerobic. These forms cannot exist in the presence of elevated oxygen. In this gelatinous, low oxygen area, they are able to do their damage. Koch also demonstrated that the simple addition of high energy oxygen actually reverses this process.

Candida does not only wear down the immune system, but can predispose one to cancer, and prevent the body from repairing the damage. (Remember the inactivation of Natural Killer Cells by the candida immune complexes observed by Dr. Wojdani.)

Every cancer patient and AIDS patient I have seen had candidal overgrowths and complications. I must concur with Dr. Koch on the connection of fungal forms and cancer.

In the 1950's, Dr. Seyfarth from the Geschwulstklinik (Tumor Clinic) Berlin-Buch found Candida spp. in cultures of all tumor cells examined. According to Bernhard Muschlien, a naturopathic practitioner from Wiesbaden, West Germany, the mitochondria of tumor cells are mitochondria from yeast cells capable of anaerobic fermentation processes, which have been exchanged for the oximitochondria of normal cells.

Dr. Von Brehmer (1884-1958) first described Siphonospora polymorpha (S.p.), an organism that is not pathogenic to the healthy organism but transforms to all kinds of virus-like particles, rod-like bacteria, budding yeast-forms and molds in an immunodepressed host organism.

Histoplasmosis caused by Histoplasma capsulatum is a similar case in point. And so is the pleomorphism of Progenitor Cryptocides (P.C.) as described by Virginia Livingston-Wheeler. Muschlien explains the tumor state of the cancer disease as a hypomycosis which is derived from Candida Albicans which in turn may be derived from Siphonospora polymorpha.

Dr. Hans A. Nieper points out that the main change of a normal cell into a cancer cell takes place on the membranes of mitochondria and microsomes which may become "autonomous" and spread via the blood circulation. These autonomous organelles, called extracellular or subcellular oncogenic agents, are derived from fungus-like structures. These show fungal characteristics in culture media.

These organells act as transmitters or messengers of the cancerogenic information to the healthy cell. The extracellular organelles destroy the erythrocytes (causing a reduced RBC life-span in cancer patients) and impair the metabolism of the entire organism (producing the cachexia of the cancer patient).

THE CONNECTION OF CANDIDA ALBICANS AND CANCER

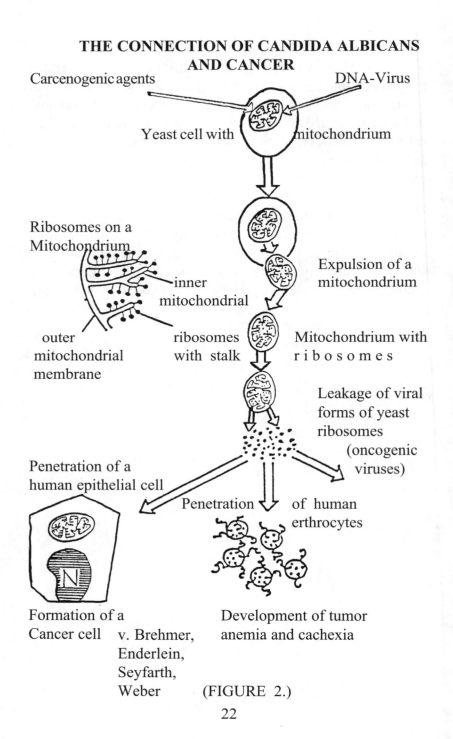

Carcenogenic agents

DNA-Virus

Yeast cell with mitochondrium

Ribosomes on a Mitochondrium

inner mitochondrial

Expulsion of a mitochondrium

outer mitochondrial membrane

ribosomes with stalk

Mitochondrium with r i b o s o m e s

Leakage of viral forms of yeast ribosomes (oncogenic viruses)

Penetration of a human epithelial cell

Penetration of human erthrocytes

Formation of a Cancer cell

v. Brehmer, Enderlein, Seyfarth, Weber

Development of tumor anemia and cachexia

(FIGURE 2.)

In 1960, Vernon T. Riley D.Sc., then at the Sloan Kettering Institute, New York, showed that these fungus-like particles formed LDH and that a cancer would only metastasize if the blood of the patient was Riley-positive, i.e., showed elevated LDH values. American immunologist H. Hugh Fundenberg, M.D., demonstrated that 60% of the people living with cancer patients show antibodies to the oncogenic agents of the patients. (see Figure 2. A MODEL OF CANCEROGENESIS)

Dogs with melanomas on their heads cause a higher cancer incidence in their owners. Donald L. Morton, M.D., then at the National Cancer Institute, now Prof. of Oncological Surgery at UCLA and Richard A. Malmgren, then at NCI, now at George Washington University, Washington, D.C. found that 98% of human osteosarcomas were transmitted from domestic dogs. Their work was declared as "classified" and has never been published.

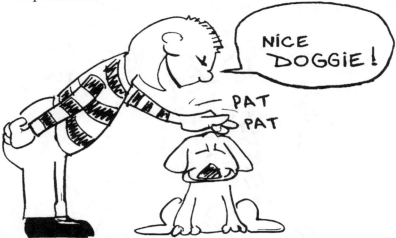

Carbon disulfide, used in the rayon industry, protects the workers from these oncogenic agents and, as a result, they show a lower cancer incidence. In schizophrenic patients, surfaces of the oncogenes (and thrombocytes) are changed and show about a 70% lower cancer incidence than the general population.

23

Toxic Shock Syndrome (TSS)

The work of microbiologist Eunice Carlson, Ph. D. on Toxic Shock Syndrome (TSS) further shows the relationship of this setup for disease. She found that TSS occurred ONLY in women who had chronic vaginal candidiasis. Dr. Carson's studies showed that a healthy woman can have one million staph germs in her vagina without any adverse effects. But in a woman with candidiasis, only five bacteria were needed to lead to TSS.

Apparently, when yeast cells surround the staph bacterium, the immune system cannot attack them. This is a symbiotic relationship that candida has with staph germs. Others are possible. With a depressed immune system, it is probable that in addition to candida, bacteria and viral attacks are being waged against the system. Candidiasis, as with all "dis-eases," is a signal from the body to pay attention to overall health.

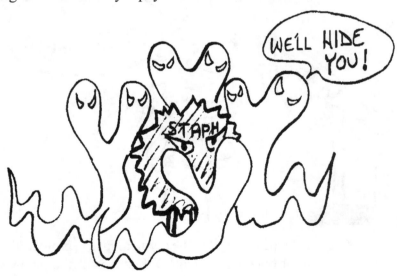

CANDIDA HIDING STAPH BACTERIA

Chapter Six

CANDIDA EXISTS

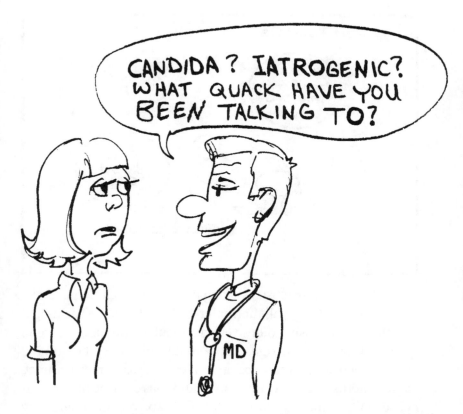

Allow me to clear up some of the misinformation rampant on this subject. Although some medical doctors are still denying its existence, Candida does indeed exist as a yeast and fungus. The medical profession calls it oral thrush, often found in the throats of babies, appearing as white patches. Candida Albincans was formerly called Monolians Albicans when found in the vagina as a whitish discharge with associated external itching and redness.

It exists in the intestinal tract as a yeast vacuole, from 2 to 6 microns in diameter, as seen under darkfield or phase contrast microscopy. These vacuoles have been microtubuled from peripheral blood samples and cultured at Stanford University. They were positively identified as Candida Albicans.

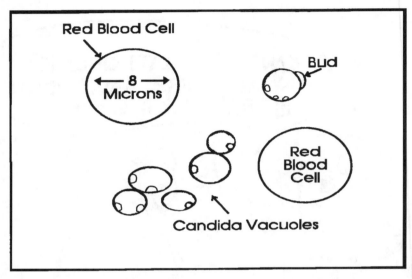

Candida also exists as a fungal mycelia which can penetrate weakened intestinal walls and enter the blood stream. The fungal mycelia can be invasive to any weakened epithelial tissue in the entire system. I have found signs of Candida to be in or behind the membranes of the ears, nasal cavity, oral cavity, gastrointestinal tract, vagina, uterus, anus, and urethra. Candida has often been misdiagnosed as Otitis media. The oral thrush has moved up the auditory canal from the throat and nasal pharynx to the inner ear. When antibiotics (ineffective against a fungus) don't work, suspect a fungus.

The term "polysystemic candidiasis" is now becoming more common in the medical field. When the term candidiasis comes up it would be wise to consider blood sugar imbalances, parasites and allergies as well.

It has been observed that persons suffering from candidiasis usually have blood sugar imbalances such as diabetes, hyperglycemia or hypoglycemia as well as concurrent allergies. Any one of these existing conditions may dispose a person to the other two. In addition there may well be a hypothyroid condition. Iodine is one of the first nutrients to be lost from poor digestion as well as protein. Tyrosine, an amino acid derived from protein, combines with iodine to form thyroid hormones. Any deficiencies here will present problems ranging from poor calcium absorption to low body temperatures, common in most people suffering with candidiasis.

And beneath all of this, the emotional turmoil, both past and present, will be doing its job of diminishing the digestive system in an effort to get attention. This is not bad. **This is the body's way of speaking to a runaway brain.**

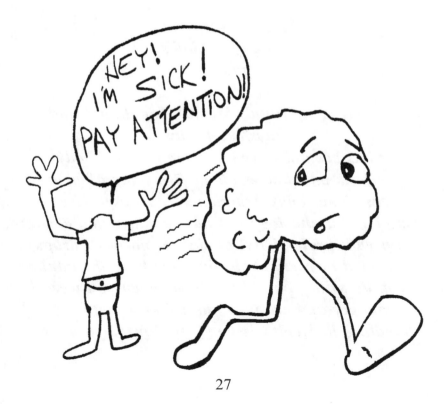

Spiritual Servant

It has been said that the brain is a ruthless ruler, but a wonderful servant. It serves the spiritual essence of life's journey by directing the loving, healing consciousness of God's energy to every part of the person's physical body that needs it. This is the only healing, the only curing that is ever done. It is done by the person's awakening consciousness. The pain, the dis-ease, the discomfort and/or the doctor/teacher only brings the person to this point, the connection between the Self and God. This is why the "whole-istic" approach gives lasting results whereas a single problem, "magic bullet" single approach, will not. By addressing the whole person, rather than the most evident problem, a real transformation in health occurs.

*There is no separation
in any of God's
parts.*

*You are a Spiritual, Mental, Emotional and Physical Entity.
It has been observed that the physical body manifests imbalances about five years after the emotional body experiences an upset. Use emotional archeology to find the cause and clean it up with professional guidance, not with drugs, sex, food or rock n roll. You now have the adult coping skills you did not have when you were younger and are now more than capable of handling it. <u>Health is Peace Within</u>, make it so.*

Chapter Seven

CANDIDA QUESTIONAIRE

Have you ever taken:
>Antibiotics for extended periods of time?
>Steroids, Prednisone, Cortisone or ACTH?
>Birth Control Pills?
>Immunosuppressants?

Have you had:
>Multiple pregnancies?
>Whitish vaginal discharge or irritation?
>Bladder infections?
>Prostate irritation?
>Erratic vision, floaters in the eyes, spots before the eyes?
>Impotence or decreased sexual desires?
>Endometriosis?
>Oral thrush?
>Athlete's foot, persistent crotch itch,
>fungal infection of the nails or skin?
>High sensitivity to chemical fumes,
>perfumes, tobacco smoke?
>Worsening of symptoms after yeasty or
>sugary foods or drinks?

Allergic symptoms such as:
>Abdominal distension, bloating,
>clothes fitting tighter at the end of the day
>Diarrhea and/or constipation
>PMS, menstrual cramps or pain
>Fatigue, lethargy, poor memory,
>mood swings, spaciness
>Cravings for sweets, breads, cheeses,
>vinegars or alcohol
>Unaccountable muscle aches, tingling,
>numbness, burning swollen and aching joints

CANDIDA PATHWAYS

NORMAL

Entry Organ:	Inhibited by:
Nose/Mouth ⇓	WBCs in saliva IgA in mucous membranes
Stomach ⇓	Stomach Acid
Small Intestine ⇓	Peyers Patches/ IgA
Large Intestine ⇓	Acid pH/Acidophilus Other Intestinal Flora Biotin IgA
Excreted in Feces	

ABNORMAL PATHWAY

Entry Organ: ## Allowed By:

Mouth/Nose   Fluoride and Mercury
⇓   Suppressed WBCs in saliva

Stomach   Low Hydrochloric Acid
⇓
Small Intestine ⇐   Depressed Peyers Patches
⇓
Large Intestine ⇑   Antibiotics
⇓   ⇑   Birth control/steroids
                                   Low Biotin
ENTERS CIRCULATING BLOOD FLOW
Liver   through hepatic vein
⇓   ⇑
Gall Bladder   ⇒   from liver
⇓   ⇓

CIRCULATING BLOOD FLOW TO:
Hypothalamus
MUCOSA OF:
      Inner/Outer Ear
      Eustachian Tubes
      Nasopharynges
      Esophogus
      Lung
      Pancreas   lowered immune system
      Vagina   with poor mucosal structure
      Urethra
      Bladder
      Colon/Rectum
SKIN SURFACES OF:
Scalp   Vulva   Scrotal   Penile   Perianal   Any/all others

Chapter Eight

BLOOD SUGAR IMBALANCES

Glucose

The human body prefers glucose as its primary fuel source. Glucose is a simple carbohydrate, a monosaccharide, or simple sugar and it is dependent on insulin to enter the cell wall. Glucose is dependent on a complexed form of chromium called Glucose Tolerance Factor (GTF) to enter the mitochondria (the cell furnace). Glucose is dependent on oxygen to be burned normally.

Blood sugar refers to glucose, not sucrose. Sucrose is a

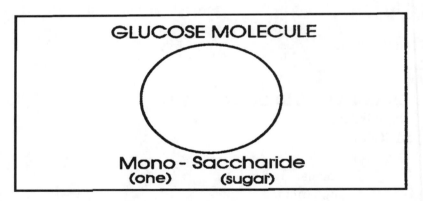

disaccharide. It burns up the body's energy and B-vitamins to be broken down to glucose and fructose. Refined white sugar is pure sucrose, devoid of any vitamins or minerals to metabolize it. For optimum health, it is best avoided.

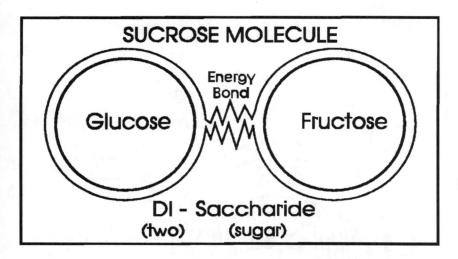

SUCROSE MOLECULE

Energy Bond

Glucose

Fructose

DI - Saccharide
(two)   (sugar)

Hypoglycemia refers to low blood sugar. This may occur if there are not enough simple or complex carbohydrates included in the diet. If carbohydrates are eaten but are not completely broken down to the monosaccharide form (glucose), hypoglycemia may occur. If there is adequate glucose and insulin, but not enough GTF or oxygen, hypoglycemic symptoms still may occur. Low functioning, stressed out adrenals produce hypoglycemia

Hyperglycemia is high blood sugar. An allergic reaction can cause a rapid rise in blood sugar, excessive insulin production, and then rebound to low blood sugar. Rapid rises in blood sugar may occur from dietary mistakes, hormonal imbalances or over stimulation, both physical and emotional. When high sugar levels remain in the blood, they displace oxygen.

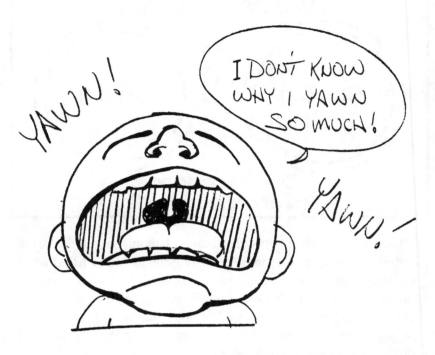

Thus, frequent yawns and gasping for air is commom.

When sugars remain too high due to a lack of insulin, it is called diabetes. If too much oxygen is displaced by the glucose, diabetic comas may occur. Some forms of diabetes are exacerbated by chronic allergic responses to foods and chemicals.

By reducing allergic substances, the levels of insulin needed are greatly reduced or removed in some cases.

It has been said that diabetes, hyperglycemia and hypoglycemia are different pieces of the same stick.

Some symptoms of blood sugar imbalance are:

fatigue	headaches
yawning	gasping for air
mental confusion	spaciness
giddiness	insomnia
increased hunger	nervousness
irritability	anxiety attacks
insecurity	phobias
depression	muscle cramping
dizziness on standing	inability to focus
spots in front of eyes	

(Please note the similarity to allergy symptoms in Chapter Nine.)

Chapter Nine

ALLERGIES

We will define allergies as a hypersensitivity of the cellular membrane to a substance causing an adverse reaction. Simply put, you will have an allergic response to any substance not digested by the body. This may occur immediately or up to forty-eight hours after exposure. The signs are indicated from an increase in white blood cells to anaphylactic shock and anything in between. Allergic reactions are capable of imitating any symptom. (See list).

Potential Allergic Symptoms

fatigue	dizziness	confusion
headache	migraines	sleepiness
aches	arthritis	gas
pain	bloating	diarrhea
constipation	esophagitis	colitis
ileitis	hemorrhoids	mouth sores
ulcers	indigestion	repeating taste
eye twitches	double vision	rashes
hyperglycemia	hypoglycemia	skin disorders
dermographia	dyslexia	hyperactivity
paranoia	bed wetting	pancreatitis
depression	anxiety	hot flashes
schizophrenia	joint swelling	sinusitis
arrhythmias	hives	earaches
weight problems	eye shiners	rapid heartbeat
insomnia	mucous after food	hypertension
middle back pain	hypotension	skin sensations
pain urinating	bladder frequency	

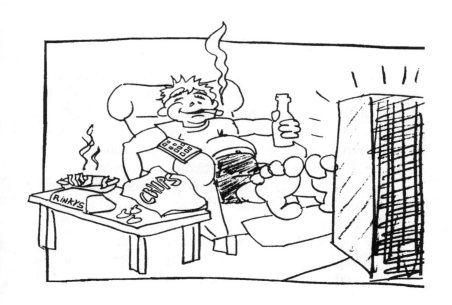

It is common to be addicted to substances to which you are allergic. Foods, chemicals, smoke, alcohol, pollens or energies (microwaves, TV, etc.) to which you are commonly exposed more than three times a week are likely to be an allergen your body needs a "fix" from. These factors stimulate people by initially exacting a healing reaction from the body. At first you feel better because of the endorphins which are released, but you suffer later and consequently crave more of what ails you. Note that most of what is sold at any fast food store chain is nicotine, caffeine, alcohol, white flour, preservatives, sugar, salt and grease prepared in microwaves among video game radiations. These are all highly allergic and addictive substances.

An addiction is really a reaction to an allergy. An allergic reaction is the inability to successfully handle an allergenic stimulus. The body is warning you to avoid this substance in the future. It is extremely important to remove allergens from the system.

The more acute the situation, the more the emphasis on removal is needed. One of the successful treatments of AIDS includes the removal of all suspected allergens. This frees up the immune system from expending energy. It provides fewer targets for the virus, as AZT does, but does not destroy the immune system, as AZT does. Then, high doses of oxygen/ozone are applied to destroy the virus. Proper removal of the dead cells then goes concurrently with a rebuilding of the damaged systems. Viral loads have been significantly decreased by using the DE Formula.

In the 1930's, a leading allergist, Albert Rowe, M.D., believed allergies were the second most important cause of disease. Currently, certain medical doctors, such as R. Mackarness, M.D., state that allergy is the primary causative factor of most medical complaints.

Allergy must be dealt with in rebuilding the health of people with candidiasis.

Chapter Ten

PARASITES

Parasites must be considered as a possible culprit. In 1976, the Center for Disease Control in Atlanta, found one out of every six Americans to have parasites. More advanced diagnostics indicate that number would now be two and one half times greater. Clinical ecologists find overgrowths of Entamoeba Histolytica and Giardia Lamblia in up to 80% of those with candidiasis. Possible signs are diarrhea, food intolerance, flatulence, nausea and cramps. In addition to absorbing human nutrients, they also can perforate the intestinal wall. This allows undigested foods to enter the blood and cause allergic reactions. Proper stool samples (rectal swabs) should be done before attempting a parasite program.. There has been a high rate of false negatives in parasite tests. Have several if they are suspect.

Parasites can be picked up from public or private toilets, doorknobs, handrails, sex, contaminated soil, water, food and dust. Improperly prepared beef, pork and fish may contain tapeworms. Pets, such as dogs, cats and horses are common sources.

A sign of parasites is a huge, swollen belly. This is not fat which is solid, it is a watery belly. There is usually great weight gain or great weight loss, anemia, tiredness and paleness. Children appear to be crabby and/or have ADD (Attention Deficit Disorder). Suspect amoebas in infantile diabetes. Chronic constipation is often associated with parasites. Limax amoeba is associated with arthritis. Programs last up to eight weeks. The **DE Formula** is paracidal and may be taken concurrently with the program.

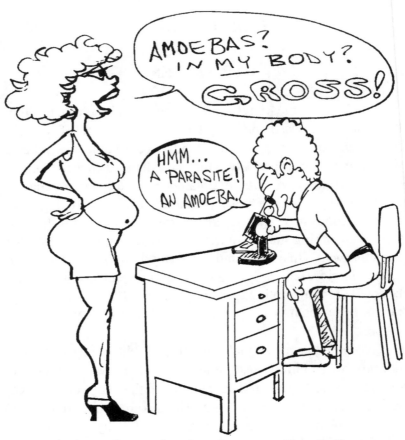

A sign of parasites is a huge, swollen belly.

High doses of oxygen in conjunction with black walnut, garlic, cayenne, aloe vera and other herbal purges (Intestinalis) are very successful in dealing with these problems. The normal production of hydrochloric acid and pancreatic enzymes of healthy adults usually control this problem. Until that time, the proper use of digestive enzyme supplements also helps to control parasites. These must be addressed before a successful candida program can be attained in some instances. Concurrent programs are sucessful.

Chapter Eleven
THE KEYS

Heal-Thy Immune System

Although some drugs and herbs are fungicidal, they do not address the underlying causes of Candidal overgrowths, a suppressed immune system.

Candida can <u>never</u> be completely eliminated!

This is because it reenters the system through air, water, food and/or sexual contact on a daily basis. The effective control of candidiasis by a healthy immune system cannot be overstated. The first key to a successful approach is control by a healthy immune system. Let me over stress this.

A healthy immune system is essential in the <u>control</u> of Candida.

A weakened immune system allows for a candida overgrowth. This is the main causative factor. Any chronic stressor such as negative emotions, fatigue, infections, poor diet, environmental pollutants, drugs, chemicals, physical traumas, amalgams, etc. will not only diminish the immune system, but will diminish digestive efficiency as well.

Digestive Support/Enzymes

When the body is no longer effectively absorbing the nutrients to supply and maintain a healthy immune system, immune suppression is seen.

41

Rebuilding the immune system is the key to *any* healing.

Because of a weakened immune system, the body is now open to an overgrowth of candida, among other pathogenic insults. It is obvious that many mental, emotional and physical stressors are lifelong influences. Until they are successfully handled, e.g. appropriate stress counseling, proper digestive support is beneficial and necessary.

Nutrients not absorbed are not only useless, but may become toxic. Even when a good diet is supplemented with the best vitamin/mineral formulas, absorption is not guaranteed. Most immune suppressed candida patients have a suppressed digestive system caused by anything from emotional problems to inherited weaknesses. Any food not completely digested will cause an allergic reaction. Mastication techniques, digestive enzymes, rotation diets and food combining successfully help to overcome these challenges.

Enzyme efficiency is temperature, molecular size and pH dependent. The proper selection of enzymes and other supplements is best preceded by an evaluation of gastrointestinal pHs.

Key two is nutrient absorption with the aid of pH selected digestive enzymes.

Vitamin/mineral

Healthy blood requires available nutrients in sufficient quantities. As a result of our soil having been so depleted, there are insufficient balanced nutrients in the food chain. It is theoretically impossible to obtain all that is necessary for optimum health from a diet of these depleted foods. In "The Betrayal of Health" by Joseph D. Beasley, M.D., the doctor quotes surveys by the then Department of Health, Welfare and Education. It noted vitamin and mineral deficiencies in over 50% to 90% of the American population eating the Standard American Diet (SAD).

Supplementation with a high quality,
pH correct, vitamin/mineral
is another key factor.

Immune Stimulation

When Candida is found only in the gastrointestinal tract or vagina, Nystatin, grapefruit seed extract, and Pau D'Arco may bring relief of symptoms in acute conditions. In chronic conditions, candida is often in the bloodstream. Nizoral is absorbed into the bloodstream, but periodic liver function tests are necessary due to its high toxicity. If a chronic condition exists, prolonged use of these drugs toxifies the liver and is not advisable. This now requires a liver detoxification program because a toxic liver also compromises protein metabolism.

Protein is the basis of the immune system.

We must first do no harm, especially to the immune system. When we do, immediately following or concurrent to the insult, stimulation of the immune system must occur for best results.

Immunostimulation with germanium
sesquioxide, garlic, vitamin C, berberine herbs ,
olive leaf extract and oxygenators
is a key that is always helpful.

It is one thing to have a high white blood cell (WBC) count, and another to have them viable and active. It has been observed too often that the rounded shape of WBCs is demonstrated in people with Candidiasis and other health problems. Although there were adequate numbers of WBCs, they were ineffective due to the lack of Vitamin C.

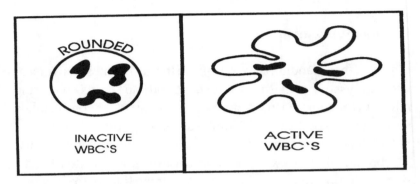

Vitamin C is essential for chemotaxis, the ability of the WBC to move toward pathogens and engulf them. If your WBC was a unicorn, its horn would be oxygen, but its legs would be Vitamin C.

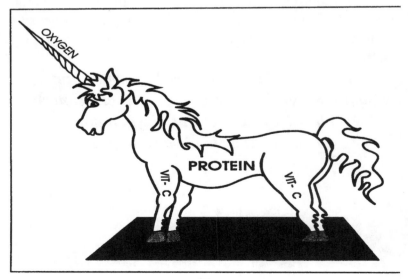

Biotin

Chronic conditions usually involve the mycelial form of candida. Mycelia can pass out of the intestinal tract, the effective working area of these drugs. Once in the bloodstream, candida may eventually enter into other organs and even joints.

In order for candida to change form, from a yeast vacuole to a fungal mycelia, there must be a biotin deficiency, usually of less than 300 mcg. per day. When this occurs, passage of the mycelia through the intestinal gut damages the membrane. This increased gut permeability allows partially undigested foods to enter the blood, thus precipitating an allergic reaction.

An allergic reaction is a hypersensitivity of the cellular membrane.

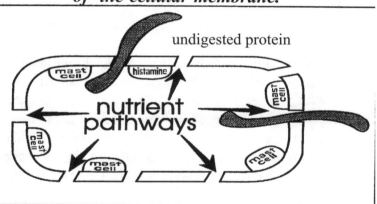
undigested protein

Mast Cells release histamine when touched by undigested protein

Partially digested proteins enter the blood through the intestinal holes made by the mycelial forms and thus irritate cellular membranes. This may be prevented by adequate biotin levels.

300-900 mcg/day is an essential key.

45

CANDISTROY

Candistroy is a master blend of candicidal, immune support-ive and intestinal rebuilding indgredients. Candistroy comes in two parts, the Candistroyer and the Probiotic formulas.

Candistroyer contains zinc tannates which bind to the candida. This prevents the candida from attaching to the intestinal wall. The candida cannot metabolize sugars and therefore die.

Also contained are volatile oils from peppermint, cinnamon, orange peel, and cloves which are also candicidal, i.e. candida killing. The essential oils from ginger and thyme have anti-fungal effects as well as the lapachol and xyloidone in the Pau D'Arco.

More importantly in the Candistroyer are the berberine containing herbs, Goldenseal, Oregon Grape Root and Barberry. Berberines are <u>powerful immune-stimulating ingredients</u>. The immuno-supportive effects of the garlic are well know. As always, our goal is a healthy immune system which elicits a natural healing response.

The Probiotic Formula is a blend of friendly intestinal floras, lactobacillus acidophilus and bifidobacterium bifidum (l. bifidis), from human sources. These friendly human flora implant in the intestines more readily than non -human sources. Lactobacillus acidophilus has the same binding sites in the intestine as candida. The higher the number of acidophilus in the intestine, the fewer sites for candida to feed. The inhibitory secretions (H_2O_2) of the bifidum are candicidal.

The inclusion of FOS and N-Acetyl-Glucosamine in the Probiotic Formula promote the growth of the probiotics for a healthy intestinal environment.

The addition of Candistroy or berberines to this program has maximized the number of successes.

Dioxychloride (Dioxychlor or DC3)

Since most pathogenic bacteria, viruses and fungi are anaerobic, increasing the oxygen blood and tissue levels is devastating to candida. This may be accomplished by ozone taken intravenously, rectal or vaginal ozone insufflation, oral homozone, hydrogen peroxide or dioxychloride. Di-oxy-chloride is not the same as chlorine. It is **oxygen** nascently bonded to a chloride ion and may be taken orally. Gradually increasing doses over four days is usually enough to stimulate the immune system and provide an oxygenated inhospitable environment for candida.

Oxygen lyses (cuts open) the outer coating of candida thus exposing it to the immune system.

Here we see again how important a healthy immune system is. High oxygen may also kill off some helpful intestinal flora. Reinstituting with acidophilus/bifidis is important to prevent intestinal distress which may follow.

Most candida dietary programs are three to six months of simple sugar deprivation and the avoidance of all yeast and mold containing foods. The inclusion of high doses of lactobacillus acidophilus and bifidus, bacillus laterosporus, garlic, zinc tannates, berberines (Candistroy), Pau D'Arco teas, vitamins, digestive enzymes, caprylic acid, olive oil, oil of oregano (P-73), olive leaf extract* (EDEN) cayenne pepper, coconut based soaps, mold free environments, and herbs may shorten this time to three months. Combined with the newer Health Guardians System, DE Formula and the use of oxygen, this is reduced to seven days in most cases.

*The most recent reports of olive leaf extract indicates its use as an immune system stimulant should be seriously considered.

North American Herbs(P-73)- Extracted Oil of Oregano from Turkey contains the highest amounts of active ingredients with the least amount of toxic volatile oils. It may also be used topically.

INTERNAL CLEANSING

The first step on the road to building health is internal cleansing of the entire digestive tract and supporting organs. This includes the complete alimentary canal from mouth to colon, especially the small intestine. Up to 85% of the intestinal villi are located in the small intestine. This is where food is absorbed, only after it is digested by stomach, gall bladder and pancreatic enzymes. When food is not digested completely, a thin protective mucus coating covers the entire digestive tract. Meals, inadequately chewed, of too much food, eaten under emotionally disturbing events create mucus. Food sitting in the intestine for one, two or more days creates mucous. Seven days a week, fifty two weeks a year, ten, fifteen, thirty years of such occurances can create a hardened mucus buildup over the sites of assimilation. 85% of those sites are in the small intestine.

Laxatives, bowel stimulants and colonics do not cleanse the small intestine. By using the 29 herbs and 13 fibers in the Ultimate Cleanse from Nature's Secret, mucous and accumulated debris may be cleansed from the esophagus, stomach, <u>small intestine</u> and large intestine. When the lungs are cleansed, the heart strengthened, the liver and the kidneys cleansed, adrenals supported and the lymphatics are cleanse, then this is true internal cleansing. It is recommended every seasonal change for the same reasons you change the oil in your car on a regular basis. A clean machine runs better, longer!

After an internal cleanse occurs, the sites of assimilation are now sending nutrients and energy to all systems in the body, espesically the <u>immune system</u>. A healthy immunes system is what heals you and keeps you healthy. <u>Heal-thy immune system.</u>

Intestinal Cleansing

With a rapid die off of candida, Herxheimer reactions of nausea and diarrhea are sometimes seen. **This is not usually seen when the colon is moving 3 times daily before starting the program.** (Note that high doses of acidophilus and coffee enemas reduce or eliminate this reaction in most cases.) Dead candida tends to become an endotoxic problem if the colon is not cleaned during and after treatment. With oxygen therapies, destroyed candida cell walls are labeled and thus phagocytized by white blood cells. They, along with ingested yeasts and molds from forbidden foods, then decompose by putrefaction in the large intestine adding to an alkaline condition. Keep the colon rollin'!!! Best cleansing results have been noticed using colonics, colemas, high enemas, herbs, regular enemas and high fiber diets in that order.

Remember that most fruit, a simple sugar to be avoided during this program, also alkalinizes the system and may also contain molds.

Anyone who tells you to include fruit in a candida diet has forgotten this fact. Fruit must be eliminated until the immune system is back in charge or supported. (e.g., intravenous oxygen drips, MGN-3, etc.).

After cleansing the large intestine, it must be re-acidified and flora replaced.

The use of whey and lactobacillus bifidus/acidophilus is advised as it does both. Without this procedure, reoccurrences have been observed. It is wise to combine some of these regimens.

49

Energy Balancing

Re-balancing the system with acupuncture and energy balancing methods (Homeopathy, SET) is advised. The immune system can become allergic to and not attack the candida. These modalities are successful in correcting this problem.

Exercise

Moderate exercise is always recommended when possible. Using a rebounder promotes lymphatic drainage and aids the system in removing dead candida cells. The increases in metabolic temperature, oxygen distribution, elimination, muscle tone, endorphins and a sense of well being are all beneficial. Hyperthermia via saunas, hot baths and jacuzzis not only aid in lymphatic function, but also induce an artificial fever. Candida thrives in lowered body temperatures. Mild fevers, such as night sweats, are a natural body response to infections of all kinds. Raising the body temperature for short periods, concurrent with herbs and vitamins, is beneficial.

Amalgams

Most silver fillings are over 50% mercury! There is enough evidence in the literature showing that mercury poisoning depresses immune function and digestive functions. The older the filling, the greater the chance of contamination. Have them removed and replaced with gold or ceramics. Some of the ceramics used now contain fluoride, another immunosuppressive agent. Some dentists will place a fluoride sheath under the gold or ceramic filling. It is not necessary. Avoid this!

Chapter Twelve

THE ANALYSIS

First, The Questionnaire (see Chapter Seven)

It is my practice to ascertain that the presence of candidiasis does indeed exist, and then determine whether or not the client has enough energy reserves to enter this program.

Note- It requires __energy__ to fight any bodily invader. Therefore, an energy buildup is advised __before__ these programs are started.

I use the standard Candida Questionnaire first. If candidal overgrowths are in the intestinal tract only, they will not appear on the darkfield blood analysis and may be absent in stool cultures. The Townsend Newsletter, Dec. 1988 #65 reports that there is a high false-negative culture rate when mucus or stool is examined for Candida species.

Seeing a sympathetic medical doctor and asking for a blood test for a *candida blood titer* can acertain candidiasis for those who wish a definitive answer.

In my experience, the Candida Questionaire at www.Healthguardians.com, is the most complete and accurate.

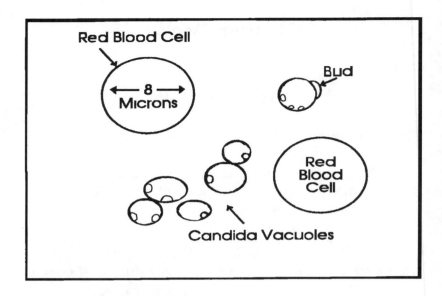

Red Blood Cell

8 ← Microns →

Bud

Red Blood Cell

Candida Vacuoles

Darkfield

When Candida has gone systemic, it will appear in the blood under darkfield blood analysis as vacuoles of 2-6 microns in diameter, or with buds before they divide. The sensitivity of darkfield analysis is better suited to expose nutritional deficiencies than standard blood panels. I have personally seen numerous "normal" blood tests from clients whose darkfield blood analysis looked anything other than normal or healthy.

The test involves a drop of blood from the fingertip, so it is not invasive. It is done within three minutes so the results are available immediately. Not waiting for test results greatly speeds up the process of getting a client on and through the program.

Urine/Saliva Analysis (NESA)

Within minutes, a urine and saliva sample (taken two to five hours after a meal) will show tendencies to acid or alkaline conditions, blood sugar problems, salt imbalances, liver and kidney malfunctions and the vitamin/mineral insufficiencies associated with those problems.

By observing the efficiency of bodily functions, sufficient energy levels to carry one through the candida program may be determined.

There exist certain patterns in the test numbers that indicate a tendency to Candidiasis, such as, high alkalinity. Recommending supplements without this form of analysis is mostly guesswork and can delay self healing. For example, it is counterproductive to give acidifying forms of calcium or vitamin C to an already too acidic person. Without proper absorption of nutrients, even the best supplements may not be absorbed.

It is essential to maximize digestive function for these programs.

High digestive efficiency also reduces the amount of allergens the body has to deal with, thus supporting the immune system. It increases available energy levels for basic body functions and elimination of wastes. When blood sugar is low from the poor breakdown of complex carbohydrates, energy goes down and the mood swings to a low right behind the drop in energy. This eventually forces the liver to release more glycogen to be converted to glucose. The energy rises and so does the mood. Mood swings are often accompanied with candidiasis for this reason.

Visual Observations

There may also exist visual signs of candidiasis such as:
>   redness of the external genitalia
>   rashes, skin flaking
>   swelling of the abdomen
>   topical fungal infestations
>   coated tongue
>   post nasal drip

The Proposal

When all the information that is available from these various forms of analysis is viewed, only then may a specific program be recommended and tailored to the individual. The client's biochemical individuality must always be considered before advice is given. Because of this factor, **there can be no one standard program for every individual with the same or similar problems**. This is another reason to have professional advice and guidance.

The ultimate goal of these programs is to build health and **elicite a natural healing response.**

Chapter Thirteen

HOW TO SABOTAGE THIS PROGRAM

It is in your best interests to <u>review this page OFTEN</u>. These are common ways this program has been sabotaged in the past. The person <u>did not</u>:

-read the entire program first

-have an alternatively trained professional

-read the labels on everything ingested

-call immediately when in doubt, or ask for help

-eat at regular intervals, avoiding hunger

-alternate foods

-have a colonic, colema, or intestinal cleaning

-exercise

-drink enough water for body size

-take enzymes

-express emotions or listen to body messages

-avoid microwaves

-avoid using "just a little bit" of soy sauce, sweetener, etc.

PART TWO

THE PROGRAMS
(Candidiasis)
(Unfriendly Yeast Overgrowth)

Many people complain of general discomfort, fatigue, head-aches, multiple allergies and high food sensitivities, often accompanied by depression and unhappiness. Frequently this is due to or accompanied by a Candida overgrowth.

The following chapter will list the primary causes and sources of candidal overgrowths. Also contained here are the main health building programs which address the methods of controlling the problems associated with candidiasis.

Please read this paragraph FIRST
before starting this method.

Most programs take from three months to one year of specific food deprivation with only limited results. On the other hand, Yeast Control in Seven Days has been carefully designed to give the highest results in the shortest possible time.

The closer the program is adhered to,
the greater the results.

Even if you believe you have greater experience with can-dida, and wish to substitute or alter this program in any way, **please contact the author or your health practitioner first.** ANY change in this program may alter the results.

56

CAUSES and PREDISPOSITIONS

STRESS (mental/emotional)

A weakened immune system (inherited, dietary, environmental)

The use of antibiotics

Antibiotics found in food (meats, chickens)

Hormones found in food (meats, chickens)

Cortisone and/or immuno-suppressants

Diets high in simple sugars and yeasts

Diabetic high blood sugar

Low residue diets that alkalinize body pHs

Birth control pills

Mercury toxicity from old fillings, or found in fish

Humid mold environments: basement apartments, showers, tubs

PRIMARY SOURCES

Inhaled airborne, ingested via foods and liquids, sexual contact and
re-exposure to infected partner.

THE CANDIDA PROGRAM

MOST IMPORTANT- Rebuilding the immune system with lifestyle changes in:

> Diet
> Exercise
> Food combining
> Enzymes
> Digestion, Assimilation and Elimination

Eliminate candida overgrowth with oxygen:

> Oral/Nasal/Aural O2
> Rectal O3
> Vaginal O3
> Topical O3
> Intravenous O3

Reduce candida overgrowth with;

> Intestinal cleansing
> Colemas
> Colonics
> Enemas
> High fiber diets
> Herbs

Rebuilding the systems that have been most adversely affected

      Acupressure / Acupuncture
      Homeopathy
      S.E.T. Energy balancing techniques
      Chiropractic

Introducing new colonies of friendly lactobacillus acidophilus/ bifidis

      capsules
      powder
      liquid
      kefir and/or yogurt

Protect skin surfaces

      wash with coconut based soaps
      Pau d'Arco based salves and baths topically
      oxygen gels topically
      internal and external use of aloe vera
      internal and external use of oil of oregano

IMPLANTS

(only if recommended by practitioner)

Bladder

Dioxychlor (DC 3)

Mix 5 drops dioxychloride in 1/2 ounce of sterile saline solution. Lie on back, hips elevated, insert 15 drops with thin plastic eyedropper, lubricated with dioxygel, into urethra while exhaling.

Vaginal

Acidophilus

Acidophilus capsules (see Natren Suppositories) or dilute Bio-K

Boric Acid

One double O capsule of boric acid powder, insert at night.

Tea Tree Oil

Suppositories every two days, then for two days place several drops of tea tree oil on moistened tampon, insert immediately. Tampon must be moist to avoid burning!

Dioxychlor Douche

20 drops DC 3 in 3 oz. distilled water and 3 oz. sterile saline solution. Add 6 drops FRESH lemon juice to acidify, do not rinse. After one hour, use a retention douche of 2 oz. distilled water, 2 oz. sterile saline with 3 tsp. of acidophilus bifidus (to replenish flora).

Garlic Douche

One quart distilled water and six cloves garlic, blend in blender. Use 6 oz. of this solution at a time. (One half teaspoon of cayenne may be used to assist garlic action).

Rectal

Coffee Implant/Enema

One cup fresh brewed, fresh ground coffee, add three cups pure water, place in enema bag or rectal syringe, hold solution in colon 5-15 minutes then release. NOTE: You will not be able to hold the solution in the colon very long if your colon is toxic. Repeat until you are able to hold at least 5 minutes. (Optional - add 25 drops of dioxychlor to solution)

Coffee High Enema

Use a size 24 to 32 colon tip purchased from drug store. Lubricate tip with K-Y jelly and insert 18 - 20 inches into rectum. Do this very slowly turning colon tip and tube in a rotating motion to prevent kinking of tube. Enema bag should be no more than 18 inches over body or fluid will enter body too fast, create pressure and be uncomfortable. If coffee does not run out, check tube for kinks. Any body position that is comfortable, side or knee-chest.

Dioxychlor Enema and Acidophilus Implant

25 drops in 16 oz. distilled water. Add 6 drops FRESH lemon juice to acidify. **After one hour**, use a retention douche of 2 oz. distilled water, 2 oz. sterile saline with 3 tsp. of acidophilus bifidis (to replenish flora). The use of whey is optional.

DAILY SUPPLEMENTS

Notes: For best results, a urine/saliva pH analysis to determine specific supplement forms (acid or alkaline) is highly recommended before beginning the supplements..

:Bottle label dosage may be checked against muscle testing for individually correct dosage.

:S.E.T. (Symbiotic Energy Testing) may be used to check for allergic reactions to supplements. Health Kinesiology Publications (415) 566-4611.

ESSENTIAL SUPPLEMENTS

High potency, hypoallergenic multiple vitamin/mineral
(_____ Mens' or Womans' Blend daily) **- supports all systems**

Digestive enzymes _____ per meal (pH dependent)
(_____ Panplex 2 Phase) or (_____ Similase) **- anti-allergenic**

Vitamin C _____ mg. per day (pH dependent)
Ascorbic Acid or Ascorbate **- for chemotaxis and adrenals**

_____ tablets HT Probiotic (NATREN) or (Nature's Secret) 15 minutes before lunch and dinner **- replaces intestinal flora**

Biotin 600 to 900 mcg. per day (Prostatin) **- prevents mycelia formation (i.e., yeast budding)**

_____ tablets daily Candistroy (Nature's Secret), or P-73 Oil of Oregano, or PlantiBiotics or DE Formula- **candicidal**

ADDITIONAL SUPPLEMENTS
(only by practitioner recommendation)
Immune system stimulants:

-Olive Leaf Extract
-Echinacea tablets (avoid alcohol tinctures)
-Whole Leaf Aloe Vera
-Germanium 132, MGN-3 and/or DMG
-Selenium and Magnesium (also for secretions)

Oil of Oregano, Bacillus Laterosporus, DE Formula - **anti-yeast**

Glucose Tolerance Factor before meals (Euglycol)- **blood sugar balance**

Pantothenic Acid 500 mg. and/or Adrenal Glandulars (Progena) - **adrenal support**

Nutri - pro, Protein, protein drinks and/or amino acids (Sea Plasma) - **supports all systems**

Fat soluble Vit-A and/or Butyric Acid - **intestinal wall repair**

Herbal Cleansers-ReNewLife, Nature's Secret- **intestinal cleansing**

Vitamins: (C, B1, B5), Amino Acids -(Taurine, N-acetyl-Cysteine), Molybdenum - **immune system modulation**

Antioxidants: S.O.D., Glutathione Peroxidase, Catalase, Methionine reductase, with continued oxygen use (AOX/PLEX)

Note - if a more detailed description of these and other nutrients is desired, call Health Guardians 1-888-231-0738

DIRECTIONS FOR DIOXYCHLOR DC 3
STANDARD SEVEN DAY PROGRAM

Dioxychlor may be taken with aloe vera juice and psyllium husks morning and evening with no distress. Dioxychlor taken with food in the stomach may produce gas.

ON AN EMPTY STOMACH
TAKE DROPS IN ONE OUNCE OF WATER

		ON ARISING	BEFORE BED
DAY	1	5 drops	10 drops
	2	13 "	18 "
	3	20 "	20 "
	4	20 "	20 "

DIOXYCHLOR may cause severe die off of candida cells (a Herxheimer reaction) with nausea and diarrhea. Should this occur, decrease to personal tolerance, but do not discontinue unless advised. The use of acidophilus and/or enemas usually prevents this.

DIOXYCHLOR may kill friendly bacteria as well. The concurrent use of acidophilus and/or bacillus laterosporus are highly indicated for best results in reestablishing intestinal flora.

Use high doses only under supervision for no longer than 4 days at a time unless otherwise advised.

SEVEN DAY <u>INTENSIVE</u> PROGRAM

This program must be administered in a clinical setting or **under close supervision only.** Detoxification of the large intestine through colonics/colemas with Dioxychlor implants MUST be done first, then followed with acidophilus implants. The higher the level of toxicity, the less Dioxychlor is tolerated. Therefore, daily intestinal lavage is essential with this program.

Dioxychlor may be taken with aloe vera juice and psyllium husks morning and evening with no distress. Dioxychlor with food in the stomach may produce gas.

ON AN EMPTY STOMACH
TAKE DROPS IN ONE OUNCE OF WATER

		ON ARISING	BEFORE BED
DAY	1	20 drops	20 drops
	2	25 "	25 "
	3	30 "	30 "
	4	40 "	40 "

DIOXYCHLOR may cause severe die off of candida cells (a Herxheimer reaction) with nausea and diarrhea. Should this occur, decrease to personal tolerance, but do not discontinue unless advised. The use of acidophilus and/or enemas usually acts as a preventative. It is also advisable to include antioxidant (AOX/PLEX) daily before lunch and dinner.

DIOXYCHLOR may kill friendly bifidis bacteria as well. The concurrent use of acidophilus and/or bacillus laterosporus is highly indicated for best results in re-establishing intestinal flora. **Use high doses of DC 3 <u>only</u> under supervision.**

DIETARY CONSIDERATIONS

The outline for this diet is basic food combining of proteins, complex carbohydrates, fats and vegetables with strict adherence to the MUST AVOID list. No teas (except Pau d'Arco) nor freshly ground coffee. Drink WATER, it is the second necessity of the body. OXYGEN, through exercise and deep breathing, is the first.

NO MICROWAVE COOKING EVER!!
(Send for Swiss Warning Microwave Article)
www.Healthguardians.com

Read the ingredients of <u>everything</u> you ingest
<u>BEFORE</u>
you eat it.

One food can sabotage the whole program.

This is ONE week only, you can do this!

Food plus supplements are essential for rebuilding and maintaining the Immune System.

MUST AVOID

Sweets:

ANY fruits	fruit juices	root beer
sodas	molasses	maple syrups
honey	Aspartame	NutraSweet
sweet potatoes	yams	cooked beets
cooked carrots	carrot juice	

White sugar and anything made with it

Sprouts: any (may be cleaned of molds with DC3 Spray)

White flour products: any

Processed foods:

smoked foods	hydrogenated

Fermented foods:

soy sauce	tofu	tempi
sauerkraut	pickles	malt beverages
malted foods	alcohol (wine)	

Yeasts:

Brewers	Bakers	bread
(beer)	(use yeast free/sugar free breads)	

Fungus:

cheese	mushrooms	peanuts
peanut butter	**raw** nuts	**ground** coffee
herb teas	(except Pau d'arco)	citric acid

Toothpaste:

with sweetener and/or Fluoride (use baking soda)

Cortisone and immunosuppressant drugs

INCLUDE FOR BEST RESULTS

3 Lactobacillus Acidophilus- twice a day,
15 minutes **before** lunch and dinner
Study *"The Digestion Digest Manual"*
Digestive enzymes with meals (HCL, bile salts, pancreatic). You will have an allergic reaction to <u>any food not digested</u> completely. Allergic reactions may raise blood sugar feeding a candida overgrowth. Then as the blood sugar is lowered by excess insulin production, a candida die off may occur with a Herxheimer reaction and a low blood sugar rebound.

THREE cloves of garlic daily, swallow whole, breakfast, lunch dinner.

TWO tablespoons of olive oil daily.

<u>TO STEAM FOODS:</u> (optional) place one tablespoon of olive oil and one crushed clove of garlic in the water at the base of the steamer for added flavor.

<u>SALAD DRESSING</u>- (<u>carry with you</u>) place a crushed clove of garlic in olive oil with cayenne pepper and use lemon juice in place of vinegar. Other oils may be used for variety, but do not have the anti-candida effect of olive oil. Combinations are allowed.

<u>NEVER</u> go hungry, always carry an emergency snack with you.

<u>SNACKS</u>: **toasted** (<u>buttered</u>) rice cakes, chicken, turkey, fish, <u>roasted</u> nuts, <u>buttered</u> popcorn, pure corn chips, plain yogurt with flax oil and <u>pure</u> vanilla (remember to take enzymes with large snacks).

SEVEN DAY MEAL SUGGESTIONS

(Counseled substitutions only)

* Suggestions may be alternated to fit your schedule.

* Use 3 drops of DC3 or H202 per quart of milk if used.

* Use your own discretion on the quantity of food you eat, but **eat at least three times a day,** drink adequate water and exercise!

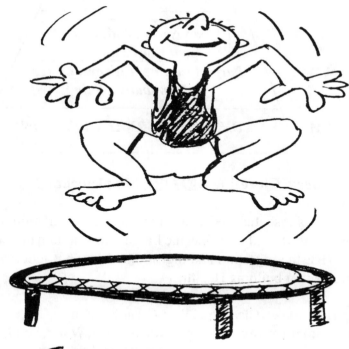

EXERCISE:
1ST RULE OF NUTRITION

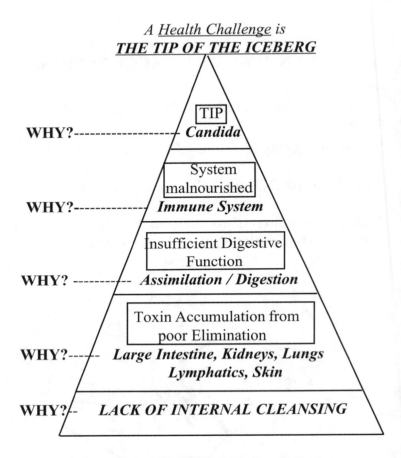

A _Health Challenge_ is
THE TIP OF THE ICEBERG

WHY?-------------------- TIP _Candida_

WHY?-------------- System malnourished _Immune System_

WHY? ----------- Insufficient Digestive Function _Assimilation / Digestion_

WHY?----- Toxin Accumulation from poor Elimination _Large Intestine, Kidneys, Lungs Lymphatics, Skin_

WHY?-- _LACK OF INTERNAL CLEANSING_

Key : **Cleansing BEFORE Supplementing**

It is essential to Cleanse the sites of <u>assimilation</u> in the Stomach, the Small Intestine, the Large Intestine, and the Lungs **BEFORE** the ingestion and digestion of Any nutrient may be optimized for building Health.

Step 1. **Cleanse**: Cleanser, Fiber, Oil and enzymes.
Step 2. **Balance**: Multi Vitamin/Mineral, Air, Water, Food,
　　　　　　　　　　B-complex, Vitamin C and enzymes
Step 3. **Control**: Dioxychlor, Candistroy, DE Formula,
　　　　　　　　　Oil of Oregano, Olive Leaf Extract

INTERNAL CLEANSE
What is a cleanse?
Cleansing is the removal of any substance that interferes with the optimum function of an organ or a system. Specifically, years of accumulated mucus covering the <u>entire</u> digestive tract, from mouth to anus must be removed.
Why do a cleanse?
When this mucus is removed, the effectiveness of the *YEAST CONTROL in SEVEN DAYS PROGRAM* is <u>maximized.</u> The building of the immune system is accelerated and die-off (Herxheimer) reactions are <u>minimized.</u>
How is a cleanse done?
The safe, quick and effective way to cleanse is to use herbal cleansers and/or vegetable juice fasting.

1. Clean up your diet by following the Menus, pg. 73.
2. Drink adequate water .
3. *CLEANSE PROGRAM* twice daily, pg 72.

Who needs to cleanse?
Most people who breathe the air, drink public water or eat commercially prepared foods, grown and processed with the above, will benefit from a cleanse.
Who should not do this cleanse?
Those in extremely weakened conditions from stress, surgery, medications, etc., should seek professional advice.
How often should one cleanse?
Every change of the season for most people.
How long does a cleanse take?
Depending on how much mucus has accumulated and for how long it has been there, everyone will take a different amount of time. Most cleanses are anywhere from one week to six months .

See **What's Next** page 82, **"The Cleanse Cookbook"** by Christine Dreher for additional cleansing.

THE ULTIMATE CLEANSE PROGRAM
by Nature's Secret

<u>Step **One**-</u> Take one tablet of the Herb and one tablet of the Fiber in the morning. Repeat again that evening.

<u>Step **Two**-</u> Increase the doses of the Herb and Fiber by one tablet each, every day until you are experiencing two to three bowel movements per day.

<u>Step **Three**-</u> After a period of time, you will notice loose stools. Decrease the dose by one tablet of each, day by day until firm stools are achieved.

<u>**WATER:**</u> It is imperative that you drink 6- 10 glasses of water per day according to your body requirements.

<u>**FIBER:**</u> one tablespoon of Fiber, twice, is recommended for those who find it difficult to eat vegetables and salads for lunch and dinner.

<u>**OIL:**</u> Two EFA Oil capsules per meal is recommended for those who have a chronic "sluggish" bowel with one or less bowel movements per day.

<u>**Super Cleanse: For**</u> extra strength take <u>with</u> the Ultimate Cleanse.
VARIATIONS
If stools are loose and too frequent decrease the fiber and the herb.
If stools are firm and too frequent maintain herb and decrease fiber.
If stools are loose but infrequent increase fiber and decrease herb.
If stools are firm but infrequent maintain fiber and increase herb.

NOTE: Use Dr. Shultz's Cleansers for a stronger cleanse and The ReNewLife Cleanse for a more gentle cleanse.(see Sources)

DAY 1

Dioxychlor on empty stomach (see directions)

Breakfast

        Cleanser / Fiber with liquid (no fruit juice)
        water/herbal tea (Pau d' Arco)
        any grain (oatmeal, millet, buckwheat, brown rice)
        <u>with</u> yeast free toast, raw butter &/or flax oil
        daily supplements **after all meals**

wait two hours-DE Formula on an empty stomach

Snack <u>roasted</u> almonds, cashews, rice cakes <u>with</u> butter, etc.

Take Probiotic 15 minutes before

Lunch

        vegetable combo (mixed steamed vegies)
        steamed, baked or broiled fish with lemon/garlic
        combination salad with olive oil, lemon, cayenne

Snack

        vegetable juice or soup with protein powder
      (spirulina) or Yeast Free Protein Plus (Progena)

Take Probiotic 15 minutes before

Dinner

        Baked squash, steamed vegies- zucchini, summer
        squash, with butter or olive oil
        celery, raw vegie sticks & avocado dip 'n' chips
        combo salad with homemade dressing pg. 68

wait two hours-DE Formula on an empty stomach

Snack buttered airblown popcorn (no microwave)
        Cleanser / Fiber with liquid
          * dioxychlor immediately before bed *

Day 2

Dioxychlor (see directions)

       Cleanser / Fiber in water (aloe or vege juice, no fruit juices)
Breakfast
       water/herbal teas (Pau d'Arco only)
       poached eggs with minced garlic,
       zucchini and onions on oiled spaghetti squash
       daily supplements **after all meals**
wait two hours-DE Formula on an empty stomach

Snack cup of plain yogurt with flax oil and pure vanilla

       Take Probiotic 15 minutes before
Lunch
       steamed asparagus with raw butter,
       Bragg's Amino Acids, baked garlic chicken (no hormones)
       vegie salad with olive oil, lemon/lime juice,
       cayenne pepper

Snack
       vegie cocktail with (Yeast Free Protein Plus- Progena)

       Take Probiotic 15 minutes before
Dinner
       baked potato (small) <u>with</u> butter- <u>no sweet potatoes!</u>
       blanched chard and steamed onions with butter/salt/
       cayenne and a combo salad and dressing (see pg. 68)
wait two hours-DE Formula on an empty stomach

Snack Fiber / Cleanser w/liquid (water, plain kefir, vege juice)

       * dioxychlor immediately before bed *

Day 3

Dioxychlor (see directions)

Fiber with liquid (vegie or aloe juice)

Breakfast
water/herbal teas, buckwheat pancakes
(Arrowhead Mills) with butter and yogurt
daily supplements **after all meals**

wait two hours-DE Formula on an empty stomach

Snack juice and protein powder

Take Probiotic 15 minutes before
Lunch
pasta/beans, vegetables, combo salad / dressing pg. 68
yeast free bread (Rudolph's Rye Bread)

Snack
fresh vegie juice- spinach, celery, cucumber, etc.
(<u>avoid</u> or dilute carrot juice, high in sugar)

Take Probiotic 15 minutes before
Dinner
steamed/baked/or broiled fish,
steamed broccoli, onions, celery with
butter, salt, cayenne
combo salad and dressing pg. 68

wait two hours-DE Formula on an empty stomach
Snack Fiber with cup of plain yogurt and flax oil

* dioxychlor immediately before bed *

Day 4

Dioxychlor (see directions)

    Fiber / Cleanser with liquid (vegie or aloe juice)

Breakfast
    water/herbal teas
    a grain cereal with yeast free toast, butter,
    Bragg's Amino Acids, daily supplements
wait two hours-DE Formula on an empty stomach

Snack   rice cakes <u>with</u> butter or flax oil

          Take Probiotic 15 minutes before
Lunch
    hamburger, vegieburger, or turkey burger patty
    steamed vegetable with olive oil, galric, salt, cayenne
    combo salad, supplements

Snack   vegie juice- cucumber (no carrot or beet juice)

          Take Probiotic 15 minutes before
Dinner
    Basmati rice, adzuki beans, steamed vegies,
    green salad, supplements
wait two hours-DE Formula on an empty stomach

Snack glass of nut milk or favorite liquid
    with Fiber/ Cleanser (if milk, use 4 drops of dioxychlor)

      * dioxychlor immediately before bed *
      <u>**last time for dioxychlor**</u>

DAY 5

You have killed off large amounts of Candida. It is important to clean them from your large intestine to reduce toxicity. A colonic, colema, or several high enemas with dioxychlor at this point will do this. Remember to always re-institute intestinal and/or vaginal pHs with whey and acidophilus implants when using oxygen/colon/vaginal health hygiene.

Continued use of **Candistroy**, two times daily is recommended at this point. The use of a DC3/aloe drink with your morning and evening psyllium, is an excellent way of oxygenating the system on an occasional basis. When using oxygen on a daily basis, it is wise to also use antioxidants and acidophilus at mid-day and evening.

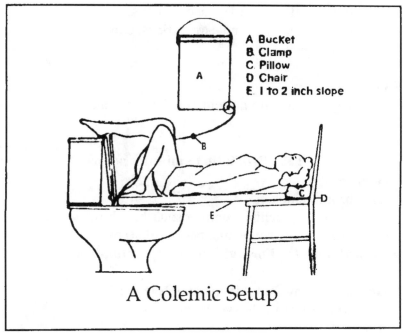

A Bucket
B. Clamp
C. Pillow
D Chair
E. I to 2 inch slope

A Colemic Setup

Day 5

Fiber with liquid (water, vegie or aloe juice)

Breakfast
water/herbal teas
oatmeal with yeast free toast, butter,
Bragg's Amino Acids, supplements, **Candistroy**

wait two hours-DE Formula on an empty stomach

Snack (<u>roasted</u> nuts) cashews or almonds

Take Probiotic 15 minutes before
Lunch
baked beans (no sweeteners) in sourdough
bread loaf, steamed spinach/onions,
sliced cucumber and carrot sticks, combo salad,
supplements

Snack
vegie juice with protein powder (Progena)

Take Probiotic 15 minutes before
Dinner
broiled chicken,
steamed zucchini, summer squash, yellow squash,
green salad, supplements, **Candistroy**
wait two hours-DE Formula on an empty stomach

Snack glass of raw milk, kifir or favorite liquid
with Fiber (use dioxychlor in milk)

Day 6

Fiber with liquid

Breakfast
water/herb tea
oatmeal waffles (yeast free) and tahini/butter
supplements and **Candistroy**

wait two hours-DE Formula on an empty stomach

Snack
yogurt, Granny Smith Apple (only Granny Smith)

Take Probiotic 15 minutes before
Lunch
any protein with vegies and a salad

Snack
glass of vegie juice

Take Probiotic 15 minutes before
Dinner
cauliflower, chard and peas
brown rice with garlic, yeast free toast
combo salad with dressing pg.68
supplements and **Candistroy**

wait two hours-DE Formula on an empty stomach

Snack
glass of liquid with Fiber

Day 7

Fiber and liquid

Breakfast
herb tea, cooked grain cereal, with
Bragg's Amino Acids,
yeast free toast and butter
supplements and **Candistroy**

wait two hours-DE Formula on an empty stomach

Snacks nuts (<u>roasted</u>)

Take Probiotic 15 minutes before
Lunch
whole wheat pasta, homemade sauce (no cheese)
combo salad with olive oil, cayenne, and garlic

Snacks
toasted rice cakes and butter &/or flax oil

Take Probiotic 15 minutes before
Dinner
Coleman Ranch Steak (hormone free meats)
steamed vegetables
combo salad with dressing
supplements and **Candistroy**

wait two hours- DE Formula on an empty stomach

Fiber with liquid,
if milk (use dioxychlor)

Day 8

A regular food combining diet.

  <u>Gradually</u> re-introduce fruits to diet.

  <u>Be gentle</u> with yourself with fruit at first.

  Candistroy is advised for the next few weeks.

  Garlic, oil of oregano and / or Olive Leaf Extract daily.

  Aloe and low oxygen drinks may be included.

NOTE: If you still feel "yeasty" after having a piece of fruit, or if you do not think it is all gone, <u>trust your feelings</u>. An additional darkfield blood test may confirm this. Go back to day one and continue the next recommended program by your consultant for one more week.

Remember, your Immune System is what keeps Candida under control. Nurture and nourish it well.

Using food and supplements, you have just experienced a "cure" of the "symptoms" collectively known as "candidiasis". <u>The complete healing involves Spiritual and Mental/Emotional work.</u> It is my understanding that the imbalances on these levels are the factors which weaken the body. Only a weakened body succumbs to "dis-ease" (see CHAPTER 2). Continue on with other cleanses.

Healing is the self care done consciously on spiritual, mental/emotional and physical levels.

Healing is inherent to the human body because health is the natural state of the Being. *"Health is Peace Within"*.

Heal thy self.

The journey of ten thousand miles begins with a single step.

BE WELL.

WHAT'S NEXT?

Health Returns in Cycles

Getting <u>control</u> over your body's health systems can and does occur in one week. Once you have gained control, the journey to optimal health still takes time. **You are not there yet,** just back in the driver's seat. Continue to feed your Immune System!!!!!

The amount of accumulated lifestyle damage differs from person to person as well as where it accumulated. If one system required cleansing, because all systems are interconnected, it is safe to assume other systems need support and cleansing. Look next to liver, kidneys, lymphatics, lungs, circulatory and endocrine systems.

Cleansing all the body's systems, Spiritual, Mental, Emotional and Physical, to where there is a free flow of Divine energy and healthy, bodily fluids is the **final key** to vibrant, optimum health. I recommend internal cleansing at every change of season.

Cleansing Can Be Tasty

The best way to health is through clean air, water and food. <u>After</u> the Seven Day program gives you control, **continue on** to vibrant health by cleansing and enjoying with recipes from *"The Cleanse Cookbook"* by Christine Dreher. **ISBN 0-9658687-7-X** **NOTE-** <u>Do not use</u> any recipes that have Must Avoid ingredients listed on page 67 if back on the Seven Day Yeast Control Program.

The recipes in "The Cleanse Cookbook" are healthy, tasty and fun to use on your journey to vibrant health. We all have to breath, drink water and eat. You may as well learn to do it correctly in your best interests. Enjoy!!!

To order call 1-877-673-0224 or email her at **seechristine@earthlink.net** or see her website at **www.TransformYourHealth.com.**

SOURCES

Dr. Sal D'Onofrio, DN, DD   1-888-231-0738
The Health Guardians   (for phone consultations)
Email- **Natdr @ aol.com** and **www.Healthguardians.com**
pH Test Kits, Analysis and Individualized Programs
"THE DIGESTION DIGEST MANUAL"
"YEAST and SUGAR FREE COOKBOOK"
     ANY OF THE FOLLOWING PRODUCTS

RENEW LIFE, Florida   1-800-830-4778
CleanseSmart, FiberSmart, Paragone, Parazyme

PROGENA, New Mexico   1-800-545-8900
Yeast-Free Protein Plus, Ester-C, Prostatin
Euglycol, Vit-A liquid, Freeze Dried Adrenals

JO-MAR LABORATORIES, California   1-800-538-4545
Free-form amino acids

COATES ALOE VERA, Texas,   1-800-486-2563
Cold Processed Whole Leaf Aloe

COMPASSIONNET, New Jersey,   1-800-510-2010 ext 4200
MGN-3

NATREN   1-877-962-8736 ext 114
Healthy Trinity Probiotic and Gy-Na-Tren Vaginal Suppository

AMERICAN BOTANICAL PHARMACY   1-800-437-2362
Dr. Shultze's Bowel Detox Program, Organic Herbal Products,
Incurables Program and videos

SOURCES (continued)

AMERICAN BIOLOGICS, California   1-800-227-4473
Dioxychlor, Butyric Acid, Candida X (homeopathic)
C2 Oxy-gel, Micro-Plex intestinal flora

BREATH OF LIFE, Idaho   1-208-443-4089
Homozone

TYLER ENCAPSULATIONS, Oregon   1-800-869-9705
Similase, Panplex 2 Phase, Panplex 8
Freeze dried Adrenals

EDEN DISTRIBUTING, California   1-760-728-0747
Original Olive Leaf Extract

SUPERNUTRITION, California   1-800-262-2116
Womans Blend Multiple and Mens Blend Multiple

NATURE'S SECRET, California   1-800- 297-2738
HARMONY FORMULAS, CO (professional) 1-888 427-6669
Ultimate Cleanse Formulas (2 part)
Ultimate Fiber, Candistroy

TOTAL HEALTH,   1-800-283-2833
PlantiBiotic (oregano plus berberines)

NORTH AMERICAN HERBS & SPICE   1-800-243-5242
(P-73) Oil of Oregano, Oregamax, Juice of Oregano

HEALTH BENEFITS UNLIMITED   1-619-938-1671
DE Formula, Nutri-Pro, Vibrum, (Angstrom Minerals)

BIBLIOGRAPHY

1. AN INTRODUCTION TO APPLIED BACTERIOLOGY,
   P.P. Hoekstra, M.R. Jones
2. AN INTRODUCTION TO APPLIED MYCOLOGY
   P.P. Hoekstra, M.R. Jones
3. A SHORT TEXTBOOK OF MEDICAL MICROBIOLOGY,
   D.C. Turk, I.A. Porter 4th ed.
4. THE YEAST CONNECTION, W. Cook
5. THE MISSING DIAGNOSIS, O. Truss
6. CANDIDA ALBICANS, L. Chaitow
7. HOW TO GET WELL, P.Airola
8. CANCER: CAUSES, PREVENTION AND TREATMENT-
   THE TOTAL APPROACH, P. Airola
9. TEXTBOOK OF MEDICAL PHYSIOLOGY, A. Guyton
10. THE SURVIVAL FACTOR IN NEOPLASTIC AND
    VIRAL DISEASES, W. F. Koch
11. TISSUE CLEANSING THROUGH BOWELL MANAGEMENT,
    B. Jensen
12. ENZYME NUTRITION, E. Howell
13. REVIEW OF PHYSIOLOGICAL CHEMISTRY 17th ed.
    H.A. Harper, V.W. Rodwell, P.A. Mayes
14. BIOCHEMICAL INDIVIDUALITY, R.J. Williams
15. CANDIDA, SILVER (MERCURY) FILLINGS AND THE
    IMMMUNE SYSTEM, B. Russell-Manning
16. THE MERCK MANUAL, 30th ed.
17. DORLAND'S MEDICAL DICTIONARY, 22nd ed.
18. THE FINAL SOLUTION, G. Martin
19. TOUCH FOR HEALTH, J. Thie
20. BALANCING BODY CHEMISTRY WITH NUTRITION,
    R. Peshek
21. APPLIED KINESIOLOGY, D. Walther
22. OXIDOLOGY, R. Bradford
23. AIDS, TERROR, TRUTH, TRIUMPH, M. Culbert
24. GASTROINTESTINAL DYSFUNCTION AND ITS IMPACT ON
    HUMAN HEALTH, S. Paul, A. Wojdani
25. THE CIBA COLLECTION 3, I, II, III, F. Netter
26. A HOLISTIC PROTOCOL FOR THE IMMUNE SYSTEM,
    S.Gregory

REGISTRATION

Register now for **a free 5 minute phone consultation** with Sal
D'Onofrio, D. N., D.D. Receive the latest information about our
publications, newsletters, videos, cassettes and seminars. "Wellness
through Education" is our motto. Mail purchase receipt to Sal
D'Onofrio, D.N., 409 N. Pacific Coast Hwy, #275 Redondo Beach,
Ca 90277 or visit www.Healthguardians.com

Name_____

Address_____

Phone_____Fax_____

e-mail_____

86

Index

Glucose Tolerance Factor   32
guidance   1

H

healing reaction   37
healthy immune system   7
Herxheimer   64
Herxheimer reactions   49
high alkalinity   53
Histoplasmosis   20
homozone   47
hydrogen peroxide   47
Hyperglycemia   33
Hyperthermia   50
Hypoglycemia   33
hypomycosis   20
hypothyroid   27

I

Infant Formula   93
Immune Stimulation   43
Immune system stimulants   63
Immunoglobulin   8
insulin   32
INTERNAL CLEANSE   71
INTERNAL CLEANSING   48
Intestinal Cleansing   49
Intestinalis   40

K

Killer cells   10

L

lactobacillus acidophilus   46
Latero Flora   63

M

Mental confusion   2
mercury   50
Microwave Article   66

TEN TIPS TO VIBRANT HEALTH

1.Fuel your Mental intentions(goal) with energy from Spirit. **Prayer** (Thankfulness) and **"Your Movie"** (visualization with sensory and emotional overlay) CONCEIVE AND BELIEVE IT

2.**Focus on Digestion**. "Stomach is Mother to ALL Systems". See the *"DIGESTION DIGEST MANUAL"*.

3.**Exercise** is the First Rule of Nutrition, <u>DAILY!!</u> Work with a professional to determine what is right for your lifestyle.

4.**Drink pure water. (Divide** your weight by 2 for the number of ounces you require.)

5.**Food Combining** streamlines Digestion (#2)

6. **Chew** food **<u>50 to 100</u>** times a bite!!!!!!!!!! Digestive enzymes are size dependant. You only have one set of teeth and God did not put them in your stomach!!! CHEW CHEW CHEW!!

7.Take **pH determined** digestive enzymes and supplements. A NESA urine/saliva analysis for a complete picture.

8. **NEVER** use a microwave!!

9.Have a **bowel movement WITHIN 2 hours** of each full meal.

10."Not all knowledge is taught in one school".

Be Well

Sal D'Onofrio, DN D

7.Take pH determined digestive enzymes and supplements.

8. **NEVER** use a microwave!!

9.Have a bowel movement <u>WITHIN</u> 2 hours of each full meal. Seasonally do **INTERNAL CLEANSING** to attain this.

10.*"Not all knowledge is taught in one school". Study and apply what is right for you. It is your Right to Life.*

Be Well

Sal D'Onofrio, DN DD

Since yeast is passed though breast milk, use of the infant formula while on the program is advised.

INFANT FORMULA

"Genius mimics Nature"
Always check ingredients if commercial formula is used,

BEWARE OF HIDDEN MSG (SEE LIST p.93)

Include in your babys formulas:

Use raw milk if possible (Stueve's of Alta Dena Dairy)

DO NOT USE SOY MILK

use raw goat's milk or rice milk and/or distilled water

Live Digestive Enzymes (1/4 capsule or more of Similase Jr.)

Flax Oil for DHA (Barleans Flax Oil or Flora Inc.)

1 to 6 months old	¼ teaspoon daily
6 to 12 months old	½ teaspoon daily
1 to 2 years old	1-2 teaspoons daily
over 2 years old	2 teaspoons daily

Lacotbacillus Bifidis (Jarrow Infantdophilus)

Colostrum (New Life)

Liquid Infant Multi Formula (Progena)

Bless it with your Love!

HIDDEN SOURCES OF MSG

Additives that **ALWAYS** contain MSG
Monosodium Glutamate
Hydrolyzed Vegetable Protein
Hydrolyzed Protein
Hydrolyzed Plant Protein
Plant Protein Extract
Sodium Caseinate
Calcium Caseinate
Yeast Extract
Textured Protein
Autolyzed Yeast
Hydrolyzed Oat Flour

Additives that **FREQUENTLY** contain MSG
Malt extract
Malt flavoring
Bouillon
Broth
Stock
Flavoring
NATURAL FLAVORING
Natural Beef of Chicken Flavoring
Seasoning
Spices

Additives that **MAY** contain MSG:
Carrageenan
Enzymes
Soy Protein Concentrate
Soy Protein Isolate
Whey Protein Concentrate

URINE / SALIVA TEST INSTRUCTIONS

1. EAT A FULL MEAL.
2. WAIT TWO HOURS (**NO** OTHER FOODS MAY BE CONSUMED DURING THIS TIME). YOU MAY DRINK **WATER ONLY**. <u>DO NOT</u> CONTAMINATE SALIVA WITH GUM, TOOTHPASTE, ETC.
3. TAKE A URINE SAMPLE AND SALIVA SAMPLE.
4. DIP pH PAPER IN <u>URINE</u> AND **WRITE DOWN pH READING AND TIME**.
5. DIP A <u>NEW</u> pH PAPER IN THE <u>SALIVA</u> AND **WRITE DOWN THE pH READING AND TIME.**

* OPTIMUM pH READINGS FOR TIME OF DAY *

***Test Two to Three hours <u>after last meal</u>

Time of Day	URINE	SALIVA
6:30 - 7:29 a.m.	5.5	6.4
7:30 - 8:29 a.m.	5.7	6.4
8:30 - 9:29 a.m.	6.0	6.5
9:30- 10.29 a.m.	6.2	6.7
10:30- 11:29 a.m.	6.4	6.9
11:30- 12:29 p.m.	6.4	6.9
12:30 - 1:29 p.m.	6.4	6.9
1:30 - 2:29 p.m.	6.2	6.7
2:30 - 3:29 p.m.	6.0	6.5
3:30 - 4:29 p.m.	5.9	6.5
4:30 - 5:29 p.m.	5.8	6.4
5:30 - 6:29 p.m.	5.7	6.4
6.30 - 7:29 p.m.	5.6	6.4
7:30 **P.M.**- 6.29 **A.M.**	5.8	6.4

About the Author....

Sal has been studying and practicing Natural Health Technologies since 1968 after observing the abuses of his lifestyle as a musician.

He attained degrees in Massage Therapy and attended Los Angeles College of Chiropractic. Not satisfied with this direction, he studied with Naturopathic Doctors, Master Herbalists and Iridologists, receiving a Bachelor's degree in Therapeutic Nutrition. While studying with kinesiologists, he learned Symbiotic Energy Transformation. In New Mexico, he learned the art of darkfield microscopy and in Mexico, the HLB Blood Test.

Aligning with the Spiritual/Scientific approach of Nutripathy, he attained his Doctorate in Nutripathy and became a Doctor of Divinity. He has also been nationally certified as a Wellness and Nutritional Consultant.

He is a national lecturer and is heard across the country on public radio. He maintains a private practice in addition to consulting for local medical and chiropractic physicians, psychologists, homeopaths and acupuncturists. His unique blending of scientific and traditional techniques has enabled him to serve in a special way, empowering people to take responsibility for their well being. He embodies a deep caring commitment to wellness through education.

"I care about your well-being on all levels:
Spiritual, Mental/Emotional, and Physical."

BE WELL

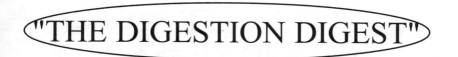

"THE DIGESTION DIGEST"

by Dr. Sal D'Onofrio, DN DD

" *Digestive Efficiency*
is
THE PRIMARY INDICATOR
in
"Health and *Prevention"*

Digestion Feeds:

- -The Immune System
- -The Energy System
- -The Hormonal System
- -The Repair System

IMPROVED DIGESTION = IMPROVED HEALTH

AN EARLY WARNING SYSTEM

Digestive Efficiency is measured by the **Nutripathic Energy Systems Analysis (NESA).** *"When NESA numbers are increasing, **Health is Building**. When NESA numbers are descending, **Illness is coming!** This is an **early warning system** ."*

Dr. Gary Martin, DC, DN.

Pouring a "pound of cure" on a symptom is *time off work, expensive, not comfortable, and **sometimes too late.*** Focus on building and maintaining your health the safe, effective and time proven way, with the Nutripathic Energy Systems Analysis.

To order call - 888-231-0731

SUGAR AND YEAST FREE "COOKBOOK"

by

Dr. Sal D'Onofrio, DN DD

A Health Guardians Publication

What to *Eat* and How to *Cook* it!

For those who "don't know how to cook" or who want more variety in their program, we offer you this book.

The perfect companion for "Yeast *Control in Seven Days"*.

An additional twenty five meals that may be included or substituted in the Seven Day Diet of the original Yeast Control book. There is something for everyone's taste.

"SUGAR AND YEAST FREE COOKBOOK" contains completely yeast free and sugar free recipes from Soup to Nuts! **What** to eat and **how** to cook it! Any meal in the Seven Day Menu is in the Index. Look it up and cook it up! Easy and fun.

Featured in the book:

> *pg. 2; kitchen cooking tips, pg 3; Products to have on hand, pg. 41 tips on cleansing, pg. 43 Daily Menus, pg 52; Sources.* $14.95 plus shipping and handling.

To place an order please **call** 888-231-0738